AF214182

Endoscopy in Small Bowel Diseases

Edited by Mahesh Goenka, Usha Goenka and Gajanan A. Rodge

Published in London, United Kingdom

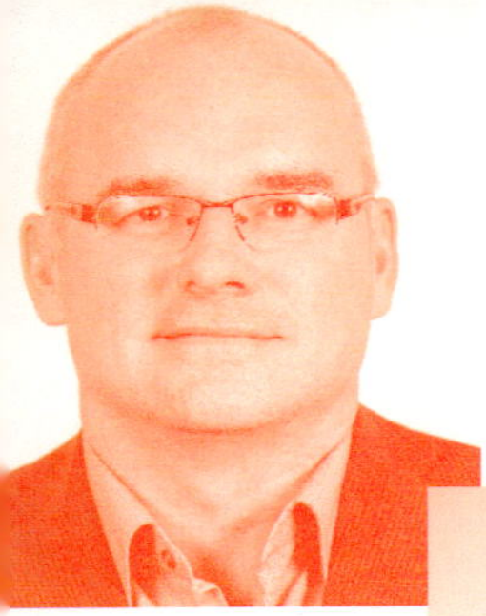
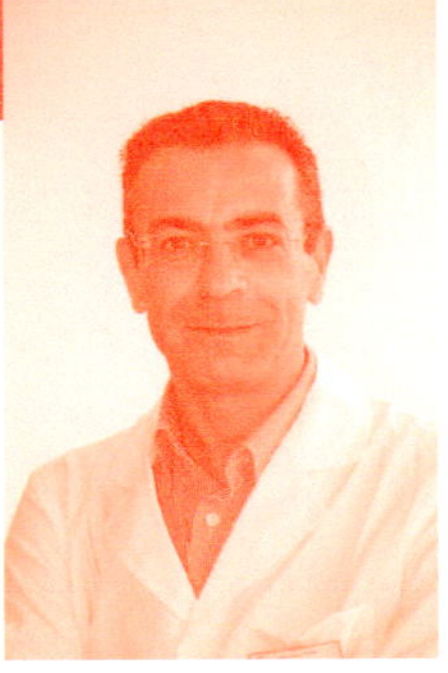
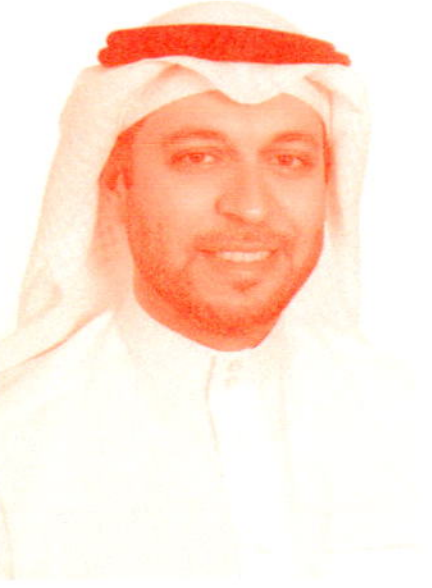
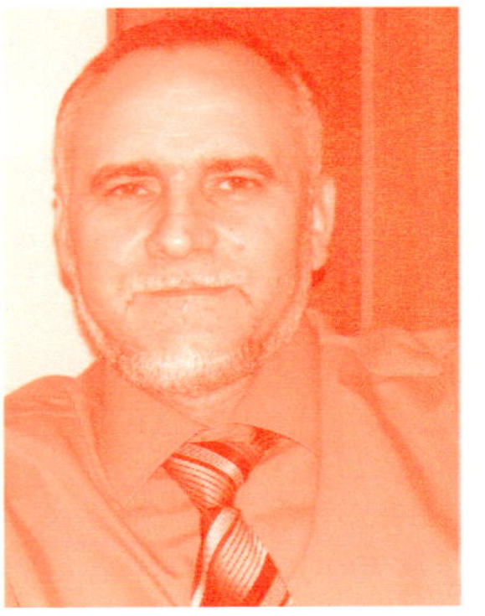
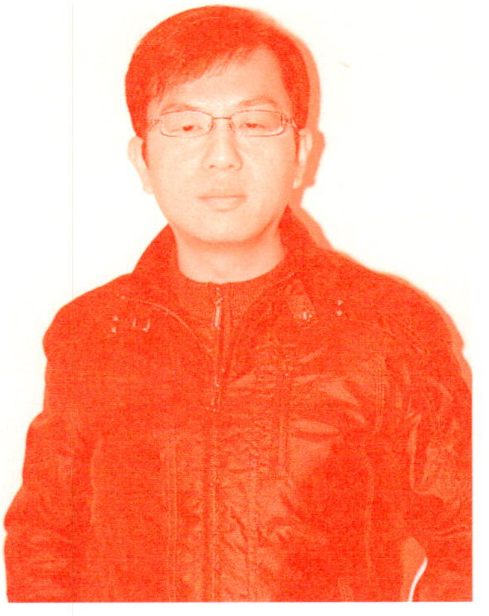
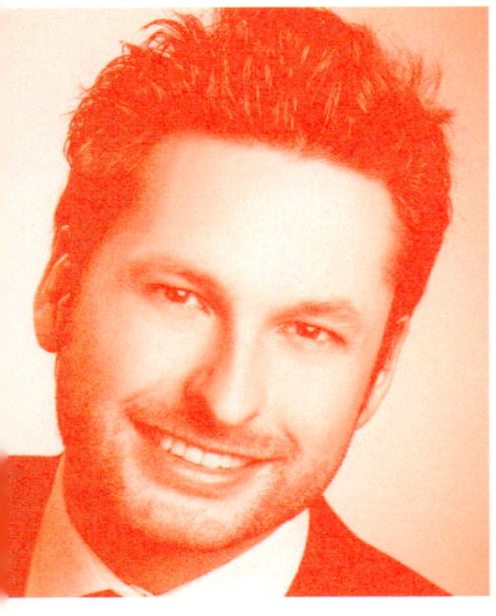
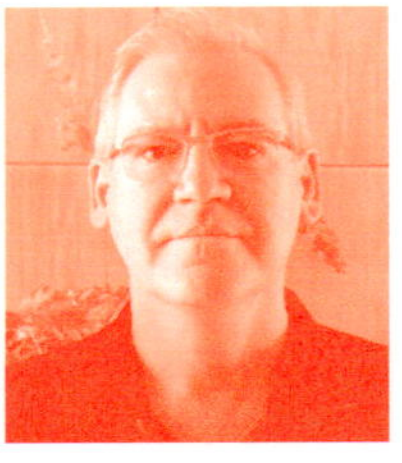

IntechOpen

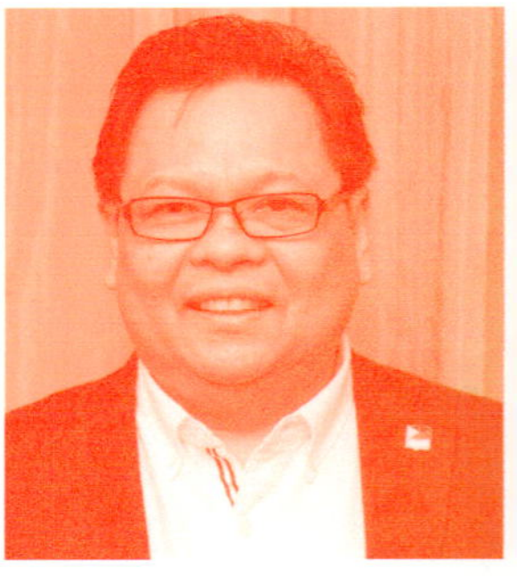
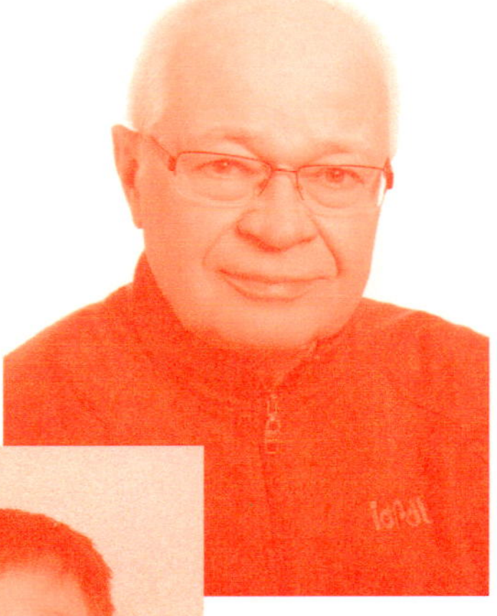
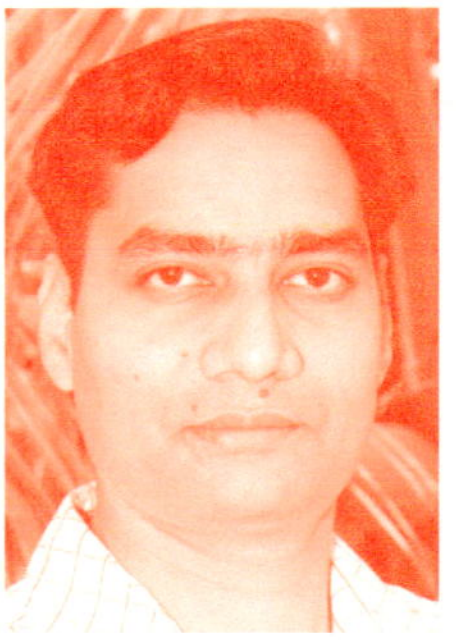
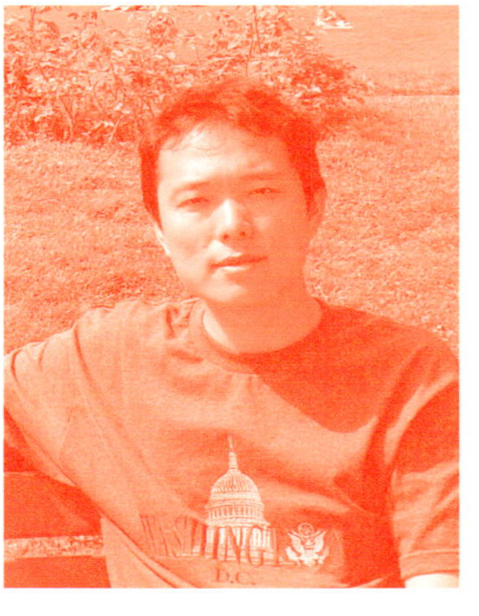
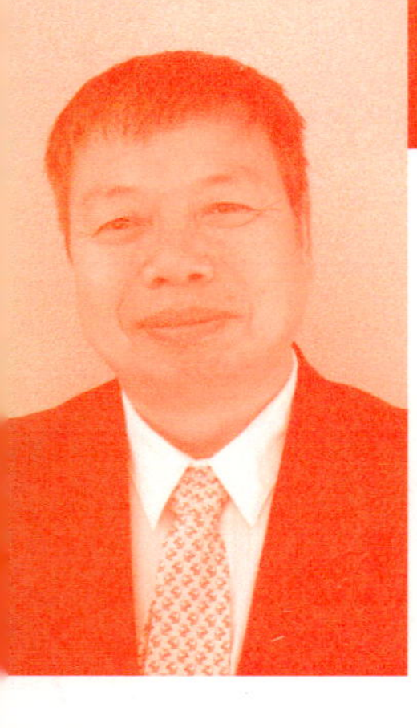
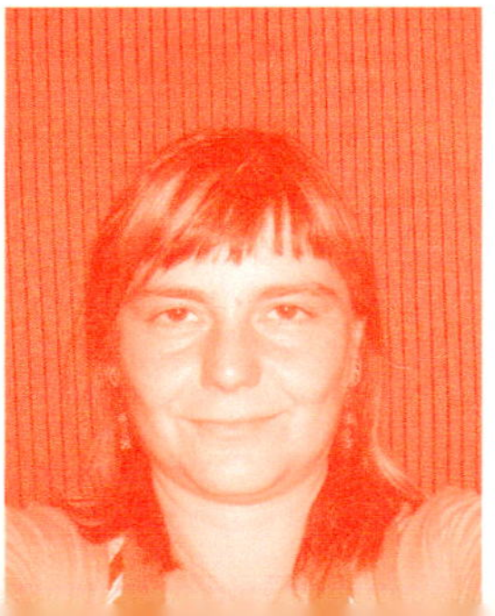

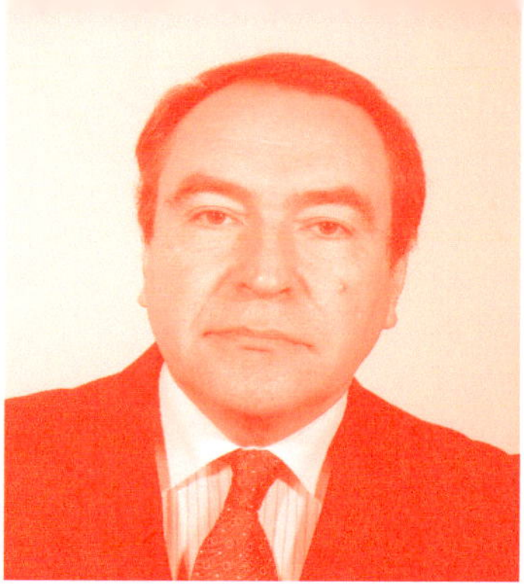
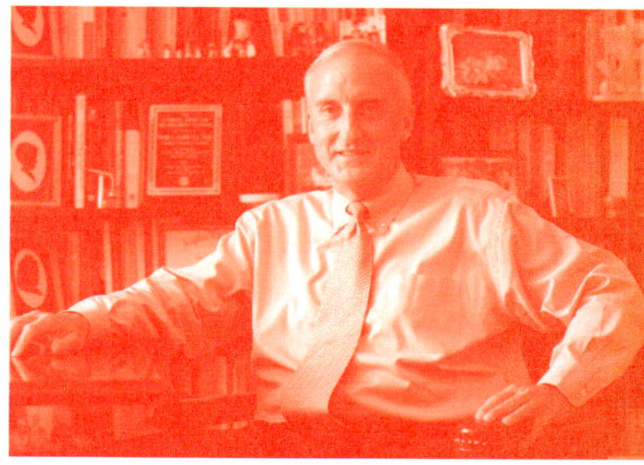
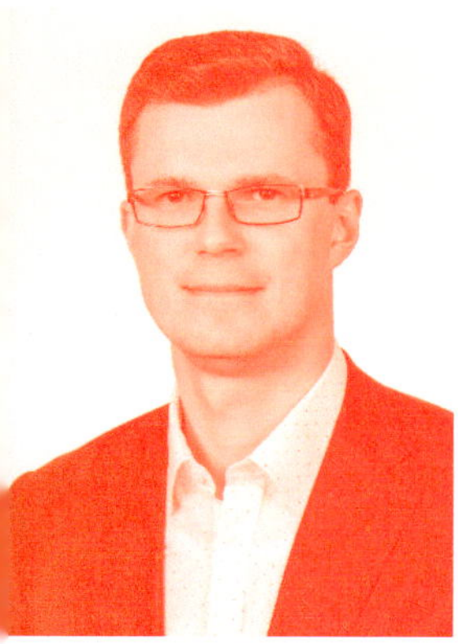
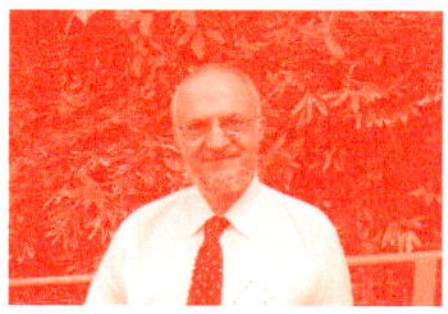
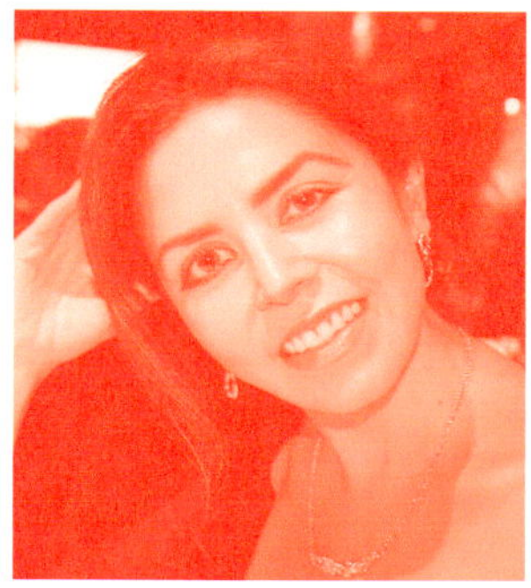

Supporting open minds since 2005

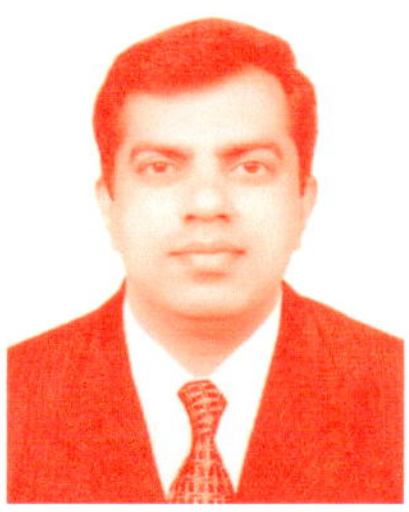
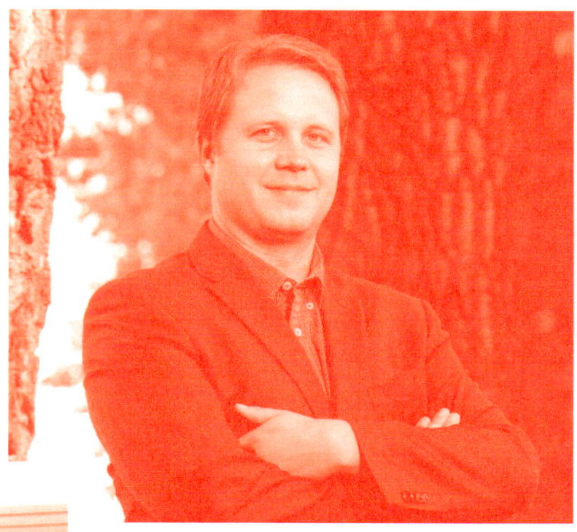
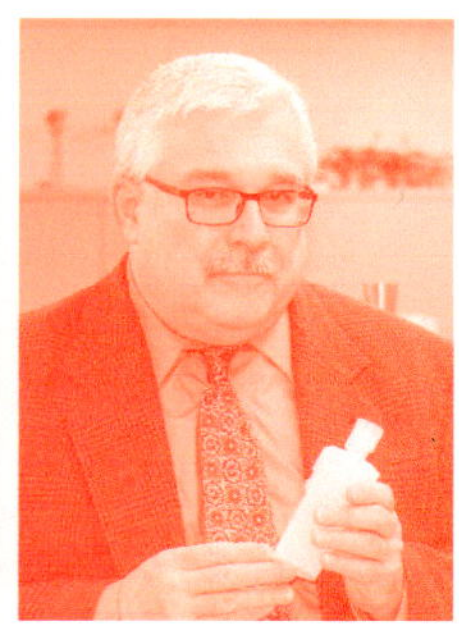
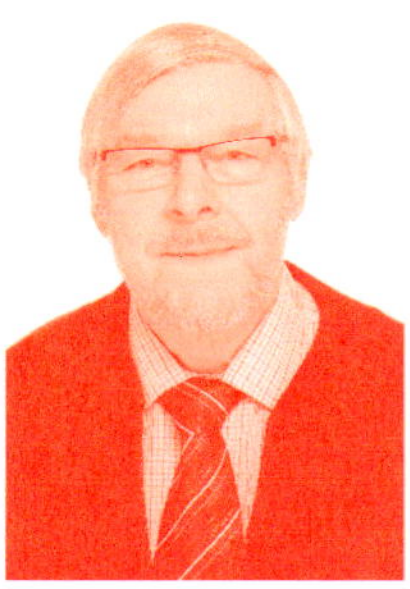
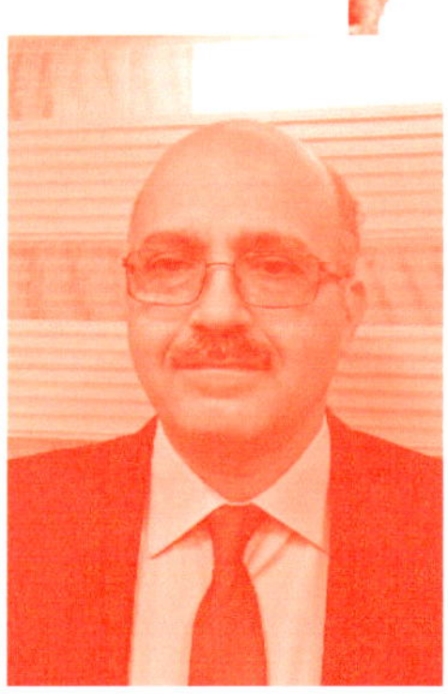
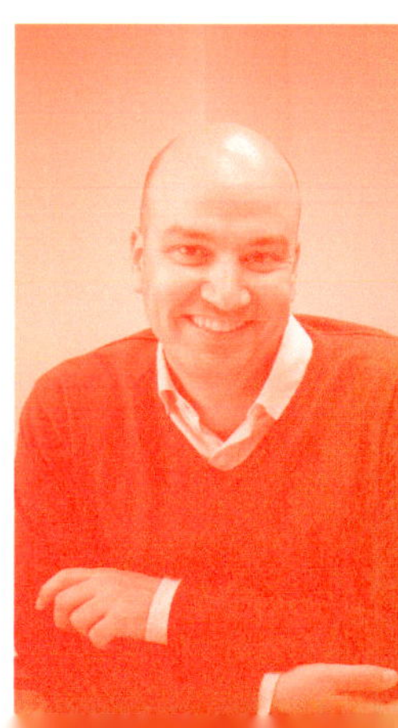
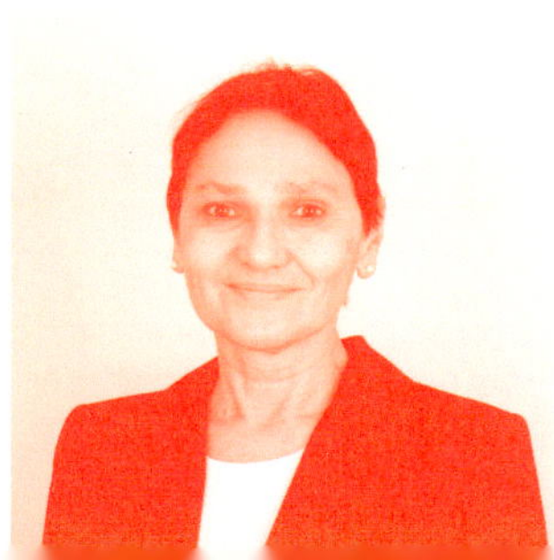

Endoscopy in Small Bowel Diseases
http://dx.doi.org/10.5772/intechopen.91495
Edited by Mahesh Goenka, Usha Goenka and Gajanan A. Rodge

Contributors
Rahul Gupta, Arvind Kumar, Jyoti Koli, Houssem Ammar, Md Yusuf Afaque, Meraj Ahmed, Noha Rehman, S. Amjad Ali Rizvi, Susana Lopes, Isabel Garrido, Guilherme Macedo, Bilal Imsirovic, Emir Gušo, Enver Zerem, Radu Seicean, Andrada Seicean, Voicu Rednic, Zaheer Nabi, Partha Pal, D.N. Reddy, Mahesh Goenka, Usha Goenka, Gajanan A. Rodge

© The Editor(s) and the Author(s) 2021
The rights of the editor(s) and the author(s) have been asserted in accordance with the Copyright, Designs and Patents Act 1988. All rights to the book as a whole are reserved by INTECHOPEN LIMITED. The book as a whole (compilation) cannot be reproduced, distributed or used for commercial or non-commercial purposes without INTECHOPEN LIMITED's written permission. Enquiries concerning the use of the book should be directed to INTECHOPEN LIMITED rights and permissions department (permissions@intechopen.com).
Violations are liable to prosecution under the governing Copyright Law.

CC BY

Individual chapters of this publication are distributed under the terms of the Creative Commons Attribution 3.0 Unported License which permits commercial use, distribution and reproduction of the individual chapters, provided the original author(s) and source publication are appropriately acknowledged. If so indicated, certain images may not be included under the Creative Commons license. In such cases users will need to obtain permission from the license holder to reproduce the material. More details and guidelines concerning content reuse and adaptation can be found at http://www.intechopen.com/copyright-policy.html.

Notice
Statements and opinions expressed in the chapters are these of the individual contributors and not necessarily those of the editors or publisher. No responsibility is accepted for the accuracy of information contained in the published chapters. The publisher assumes no responsibility for any damage or injury to persons or property arising out of the use of any materials, instructions, methods or ideas contained in the book.

First published in London, United Kingdom, 2021 by IntechOpen
IntechOpen is the global imprint of INTECHOPEN LIMITED, registered in England and Wales, registration number: 11086078, 5 Princes Gate Court, London, SW7 2QJ, United Kingdom
Printed in Croatia

British Library Cataloguing-in-Publication Data
A catalogue record for this book is available from the British Library

Additional hard and PDF copies can be obtained from orders@intechopen.com

Endoscopy in Small Bowel Diseases
Edited by Mahesh Goenka, Usha Goenka and Gajanan A. Rodge
p. cm.
Print ISBN 978-1-83968-779-2
Online ISBN 978-1-83968-780-8
eBook (PDF) ISBN 978-1-83968-781-5

For EU product safety concerns:
IN TECH d.o.o., Prolaz Marije Krucifikse Kozulić 3, 51000 Rijeka, Croatia, info@intechopen.com or visit our website at intechopen.com.

We are IntechOpen, the world's leading publisher of Open Access books

Built by scientists, for scientists

5,200+
Open access books available

128,000+
International authors and editors

150M+
Downloads

156
Countries delivered to

Our authors are among the
Top 1%
most cited scientists

12.2%
Contributors from top 500 universities

WEB OF SCIENCE™

Selection of our books indexed in the Book Citation Index
in Web of Science™ Core Collection (BKCI)

Interested in publishing with us?
Contact book.department@intechopen.com

Numbers displayed above are based on latest data collected.
For more information visit www.intechopen.com

Meet the editors

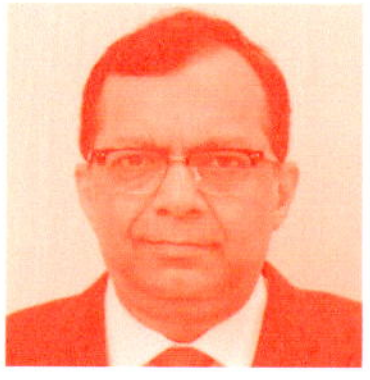

Dr. Mahesh Kumar Goenka is a senior gastroenterologist with a special interest in the field of endoscopy. He has performed more than 100,000 endoscopic procedures with expertise in advanced therapeutic endoscopy such as endoscopic retrograde cholangiopancreatography (ERCP), SpyGlass Cholangioscopy, laser lithotripsy, and so on. He is currently the director of the Institute of Gastrosciences and Liver, Apollo Gleneagles Hospital, Kolkata, India. He is also a national convener for the National Board of Examination for Medical Gastroenterology. He has more than 175 publications in various books and national and international medical journals. He was recently elected as the president-elect of the Indian Society of Gastroenterology (2020–2021) and governor (Indian region) of the American College of Gastroenterology (ACG). He also served as secretary general and president of the Society of Gastrointestinal Endoscopy of India (2016–2017), for which he successfully organized the international conference "Asian Pacific Digestive Week 2019." He is an honorary professor for the Medical School of Wisconsin, USA. Dr. Goenka is the recipient of multiple national and international awards, including the prestigious International Leadership Award (2020) from the American College of Gastroenterology for his contributions to gastroenterology in the international arena.

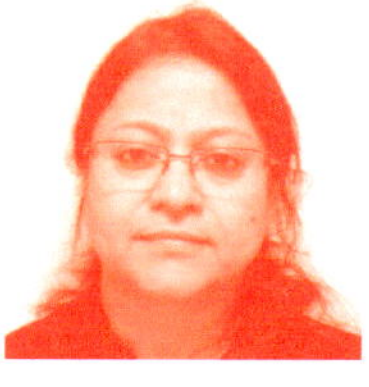

Dr. Usha Goenka is a senior interventional radiologist who specializes in vascular and nonvascular interventional radiology. She is currently director and head of the Department of Clinical Imaging and Interventional Radiology at Apollo Gleneagles Hospital, Kolkata, India. She has been a merit holder and university topper through her MBBS graduation. She completed an MD in Radiology from the prestigious Postgraduate Institute of Medical Education and Research (PGIMER), India. She has more than forty-five publications in various national and international journals. She has a keen interest in teaching and has delivered more than fifty lectures in national and international conferences. Dr.Goenka is also a member of the American College of Gastroenterology.

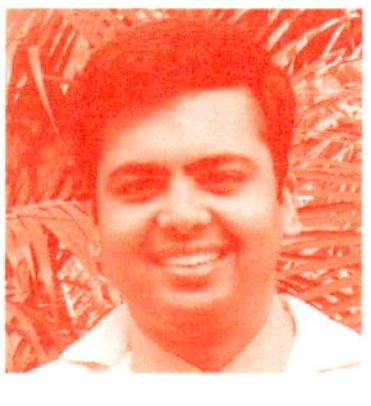

Dr. Gajanan A. Rodge is a budding gastroenterologist with a special interest in endoscopy. He is currently working in the Gastroenterology Department at the Institute of Gastrosciences and Liver, Apollo Gleneagles Hospital, Kolkata, India. He obtained his MBBS from Grant Medical College, Mumbai, and was awarded the JRD Tata scholarship. He completed his DNB in Internal Medicine at Lilavati Hospital & Research Centre, Mumbai, and has experience as a clinical associate in Gastroenterology at Lilavati Hospital. Dr. Rodge was recently awarded the "Poster of Distinction Award" at Asia Pacific Digestive Week (APDW) 2019 and the "Young Investigator Award" at the Asian Pacific Association for the Study of the Liver (APASL) 2021.

Contents

Preface

Since the time when endoscopy and colonoscopy were first introduced, small bowel disorders have remained a diagnostic challenge. The small bowel or the midgut is difficult to assess due to its location and distance from the oral and anal openings. Whereas endoscopy and colonoscopy were commonly used for the diagnosis and treatment of acid peptic, neoplastic, and inflammatory gastrointestinal disorders, the midgut remained an endoscopic mystery. With the exception of surgically assisted scope insertion through a jejunal enterotomy, entry to the small bowel was limited to the edges reaching only to the proximal jejunum or terminal ileum. Imaging modalities like barium studies and computed tomography scans were the options initially used for small bowel assessment.

The past few decades have seen many developments in imaging modalities for the small bowel, leading to better diagnosis and focused therapy. This includes the innovation of capsule endoscopy, which was a revolution in small bowel imaging and led to a change in the diagnostic algorithm for obscure gastrointestinal (GI) bleeding. Later advances like double balloon and spiral enteroscopy now provide a therapeutic option for small bowel diseases. Although this book mainly covers the endoscopic aspect of small bowel diseases, we have included a separate chapter on radiological imaging in inflammatory bowel diseases (IBD). Radiological imaging is an important complementary tool for the diagnosis of small bowel diseases.

This book reviews not only the history and art of small bowel endoscopy but also covers other aspects like endoscopic ultrasound assessment of the duodenal wall, intra-operative endoscopy, and management of small bowel perforations. We hope it will help readers in the management of patients with small bowel diseases.

Mahesh Kumar Goenka and Gajanan A. Rodge
Institute of Gastrosciences and Liver,
Apollo Gleneagles Hospital,
Kolkata, India

Usha Goenka
Department of Clinical Imaging and Interventional Radiology,
Apollo Gleneagles Hospital,
Kolkata, India

Section 1

Introduction

Chapter 1

Introductory Chapter: Endoscopy in Small Bowel Diseases

Usha Goenka, Gajanan Ashokrao Rodge and Mahesh Kumar Goenka

1. Introduction

The small bowel diseases are known to pose a diagnostic challenge for the clinicians in a day-to-day practice. Different small bowel pathologies can broadly be divided as vascular, inflammatory or neoplastic disorders. The most common indication for imaging of small bowel in clinical practice is obscure gastro-intestinal (GI) bleeding. Other indications for small bowel evaluation include Crohn's disease, tuberculosis, NSAID induced ulcers, small bowel malignancies, polyposis syndromes and malabsorptive disorders.

The routine means of endoscopic evaluation in the form of upper gastro-intestinal (GI) endoscopy and lower GI endoscopy limit the assessment of GI tract upto the duodenum and ileum respectively. The small bowel was initially out of reach for the diagnostic and therapeutic endoscopy procedures. In 1982 Shinya first reported the use of push enteroscopy and described finding of a small bowel tumour [1]. Use of push enteroscopy was later reported in different studies in the subsequent years [2–4]. Later came the sonde (French word for probe) enteroscopy which involves passage of a thin trans-nasal endoscope with a hood or balloon on its tip that is dragged distally by peristaltic movements of the intestine. It took a period of 13 years for its development [5]. Lewis et al., reported the use of sonde enteroscopy and found the small bowel bleeding site in 33% of patients who presented with obscure GI bleeding (60 patients) [6]. However due to the disadvantages as requirement of longer time, limited passage in presence of adhesions, strictures, and motility disturbances it was later found to be inefficient and lost its popularity.

Barium imaging and computed tomography (CT) scans were the mainstay of small bowel imaging till the year 2000. The innovation of wireless capsule endoscopy has revolutionised the small bowel imaging and has made its own place in the diagnostic algorithm for various small bowel diseases. A randomised trial comparing wireless capsule and push enteroscopy for detecting small bowel lesions in nine canine small bowels showed that the capsules significantly performed better than push enteroscopy [7]. Subsequent studies also showed that capsule endoscopy had higher diagnostic yield and was better than push enteroscopy in patients with chronic GI bleeding [8]. Even in today's date video capsule endoscopy plays an important role in the diagnosis of small bowel diseases. However, the disadvantage lies in the inability to sample small bowel mucosa and perform therapeutic interventions.

Hironori Yamamoto introduced the technique of double balloon enterosocpy (DBE) and showed that the double balloon method facilitates passage of endoscope to the small intestine. This advent of DBE was a major breakthrough for the diagnosis and treatment of small bowel disorders [9]. Single-balloon enteroscopy

(SBE) was later introduced in a couple of years [10]. The advantage of SBE was that it is technically easier to perform compared to DBE. Spiral enteroscopy (SE) was introduced in 2008 which was a similar technique for deep small-bowel intubation that used a spiral overtube to pleat the bowel loops of small intestine [11]. The various device assisted techniques have been compared in a metaanalysis by Gu Y, et al. [12]. DBE and SBE had similar clinical outcomes and SE also showed comparable diagnostic and therapeutic yields with DBE. SBE had a shorter procedure time at the cost of less depth of insertion when compared with DBE.

The latest innovation of the motorised spiral enteroscopy (MSE) looks promising. Neuhaus H et al., initially reported the technique and clinical use of the novel MSE [13]. It evaluates the small bowel in a controlled manner, gives a good diagnostic yield, requires less time and has proven to be safe in the published studies. The first prospective clinical feasibility study has been recently published and has shown promising results [14]. Subsequent studies and case reports have shown the use of MSE for diagnosis and treatment of small bowel lesions [15, 16]. **Figure 1** shows the timeline of development of different techniques in small bowel endoscopy.

This book will give a detailed overview regarding the different techniques of small bowel endoscopy such as device assisted enteroscopy, capsule endoscopy, etc. Role of endoscopy in diseases of small bowel such as Inflammatory Bowel Disease (IBD) is discussed in separate chapters. We also have a chapter "Role of Imaging in small bowel Crohn's disease" which discusses the different radiological investigations like barium studies, CT scan and Magnetic Resonance Imaging in patients with IBD.

The different aspects of intra-operative endoscopy and its role in the management of small bowel diseases have been emphasised in a separate chapter. All procedures have some complications and similarly perforation in the small bowel is a possible complication of small bowel endoscopy. Early recognition is the key and so we have a chapter on "Early recognition and management of small bowel perforation". The role of endoscopic ultrasound (EUS) is also now well established in the field of gastroenterology with many applications. This book includes a chapter on "Role of EUS in assessment of duodenal wall lesion".

The book has been written by experts in the respective fields and we hope it will prove to be a valuable resource for all the training and practising gastroenterologists, physicians and surgeons who are looking for a composite overview of endoscopy in small bowel diseases.

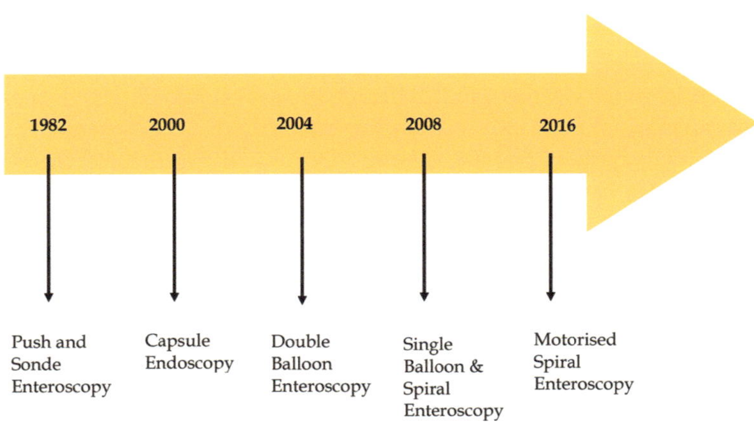

Figure 1.
The timeline changes in development of small bowel endoscopy.

Author details

Usha Goenka[1], Gajanan Ashokrao Rodge[2] and Mahesh Kumar Goenka[2]*

1 Department of Interventional Radiology and Clinical Imaging, Apollo Gleneagles Hospital, Kolkata, India

2 Institute of Gastrosciences and Liver, Apollo Gleneagles Hospital, Kolkata, India

*Address all correspondence to: mkgkolkata@gmail.com

IntechOpen

© 2021 The Author(s). Licensee IntechOpen. This chapter is distributed under the terms of the Creative Commons Attribution License (http://creativecommons.org/licenses/by/3.0), which permits unrestricted use, distribution, and reproduction in any medium, provided the original work is properly cited.

References

[1] Shinya H, McSherry C. Endoscopy of the small bowel. Surg Clin North Am. 1982;62:821-824.

[2] Parker H, Agayoff J. Enteroscopy and small bowel biopsy utilizing a peroral colonoscope. Gastrointest Endosc. 1983;29:139-140.

[3] Hashmi M, Sorokin J, Levine S. Jejunal leiomyoma: an endoscopic diagnosis. Gastrointest Endosc. 1985;31:81-83.

[4] Shigematsu A, Iida M, Hatanaka M, et al. Endoscopic diagnosis of lymphangioma of the small intestine. Am J Gastroenterol. 1988;83:1289-93.

[5] Tada M, Kawai K. Small bowel endoscopy. Scand J Gastroenterol. 1984;19 Suppl 102:39-52.

[6] Lewis B, Waye J. Gastrointestinal bleeding of obscure origin: the role of small bowel enteroscopy. Gastroenterology. 1988;94:1117-1120.

[7] Appleyard M, Fireman Z, Glukhovsky A, et al. A randomized trial comparing wireless capsule endoscopy with push enteroscopy for the detection of small-bowel lesions. Gastroenterology. 2000 Dec;119:1431-1438.

[8] Hartmann D, Schilling D, Bolz G, et al. Capsule endoscopy versus push enteroscopy in patients with occult gastrointestinal bleeding. Z Gastroenterol. 2003;41:377-382.

[9] Yamamoto H, Kita H, Sunada K, et al. Clinical outcomes of double-balloon endoscopy for the diagnosis and treatment of small-intestinal diseases. Clin Gastroenterol Hepatol. 2004;2:1010-1016.

[10] Kawamura T, Yasuda K, Tanaka K, et al. Clinical evaluation of a newly developed single-balloon enteroscope. Gastrointest Endosc. 2008;68:1112-1116.

[11] Akerman PA, Agrawal D, Cantero D, Pangtay J. Spiral enteroscopy with the new DSB overtube: a novel technique for deep peroral small-bowel intubation. Endoscopy. 2008;40:974-978.

[12] Gu Y, Shi X, Yang Y, et al. Single-balloon and spiral enteroscopy may have similar diagnostic and therapeutic yields to double-balloon enteroscopy: Results from a meta-analysis of randomized controlled trials and prospective studies. World J of Meta-Anal. 2020;8:153-162

[13] Neuhaus H, Beyna T, Schneider M, Devière J. Novel motorized spiral enteroscopy: first clinical case. Video GIE 2016;1: 32-33.

[14] Beyna T, Arvanitakis M, Schneider M, et al. Motorised spiral enteroscopy: first prospective clinical feasibility study. Gut 2020;0: 1-7.

[15] Ramchandani M, Rughwani H, Inavolu P, et al. Diagnostic yield and therapeutic impact of novel motorized spiral enteroscopy in small-bowel disorders: a single-center, real-world experience from a tertiary care hospital (with video). Gastrointest Endosc. Epub. 2020.

[16] Rodge GA, Ramchandani M, Shah BB, Afzalpurkar S, Raj DB, Goenka MK. Hemoclips during motorized spiral enteroscopy—A unique case. Indian J Gastroenterol (2020). https://doi.org/10.1007/s12664-020-01097-w

Section 2

Imaging in Small Bowel

Chapter 2

Role of Imaging in Small Bowel Crohn's Disease

Bilal Imširović, Enver Zerem and Emir Gušo

Abstract

The small intestine is a challenging organ for clinical and radiological evaluation. The introduction of radiological imaging techniques, which do not significantly disturb patients' comfort and safety, attempts to obtain an adequate diagnosis and valuable information. The aim is to determine the capabilities and potential of ultrasound, computed tomography (CT), diffusion-weighted imaging (DWI), and contrast-enhanced magnetic resonance (MR) enterography to establish the diagnosis and to evaluate the severity and activity of intestinal inflammation. Conventional ultrasound is a suitable orientation method in the initial evaluation of patients with Crohn's disease. At the same time, contrast-enhanced MR enterography provides an excellent assessment of disease activity, as well as the complications that accompany it. Contrast-enhanced MR enterography, combined with DWI, allows for excellent evaluation of disease activity and problems or difficulties following it. The examination can be repeated, controlled and can monitor patients with this disease.

Keywords: ultrasound, computed tomography, diffusion, inflammatory bowel disease, magnetic resonance imaging

1. Introduction

Crohn's disease or enteritis regionalis is a chronic inflammatory disease of the digestive tract, predominantly of the small intestine. It is the most common small bowel disease in the United States and Europe: (3.1–14.6/100,000 in the United States and 0.7–9.8/100,000 in Europe, respectively) [1]. It occurs more frequently in the White population than in African-American and Asian ones, and is particularly common in certain ethnic groups [2]. The disease is equally present in both sexes and most often occurs between twenty and forty years of age [3].

Research into the epidemiology of IBD in areas with a sharply increased incidence may discover important etiological factors associated with the disease development [4].

Although the process most commonly affects the terminal ileum (60–80% of cases), the disease can occur in any part of the digestive tract, from the mouth to the anus [5].

Crohn's disease is a disease of segmental nature, in which healthy parts of the intestine are located between the affected ones. The inflammatory process spreads to all layers of the wall and affects the mesentery and local lymph glands [5, 6].

Many patients have lesions on the terminal ileum and the colon; in many cases, it is challenging to distinguish Crohn's disease from ulcerative colitis by differential diagnosis. Therefore, for ulcerative colitis and Crohn's disease, there is a common name - inflammatory bowel disease (IBD) [6, 7].

Inflammatory changes in the early stage of the disease are more pronounced in the submucosa than in the mucosa due to lymphedema [8]. The mucosa's lamina propria is infiltrated by polymorphonuclear leukocytes, forming crypt abscesses as a sign of the earliest lesion; this is followed by an enlargement of the lymphoid follicles surrounded by a red ring. Aphthoid ulceration appears on the mucosa, which progresses to deep, most often longitudinal ulcers in the disease's further course. As the disease progresses, the inflammation spreads transmurally with the formation of deep fissures and ulcerations along with the entire wall thickness.

In the advanced stage of the disease, fibrous strictures and extramural fistulas and abscesses develop [9].

Complications in Crohn's disease are common and can be local and extraintestinal [10].

2. Diagnosis of the disease

Inflammatory bowel diseases, especially small bowel diseases, have always posed a diagnostic challenge [11]. The small intestine is a very challenging organ for clinical and radiological evaluation. Detecting the disease and determining its prevalence are two important clinical and diagnostic tasks.

In addition to the above, an important question to be answered is the degree of the disease's inflammatory activity. Although the medical issue was defined in the last century, diagnostic problems are still present. Advances in technology and the introduction of new diagnostic procedures promise better results.

2.1 Imaging techniques in the diagnosis of Crohn's disease

Ultrasound, computed tomography, and MRI are the techniques often used in the diagnosis of abdominal disease.

2.1.1 Ultrasound

Ultrasound is a widely used diagnostic modality that, due to its availability, simplicity, absence of harmful effects, and low cost of the examination, is the first diagnostic method used to diagnose abdominal diseases [12].

Ultrasound is generally performed without the use of a contrast agent. Some studies indicate greater sensitivity after the administration of an ultrasound contrast agent [13].

Technological advances and the growing experience of radiologists make ultrasound an increasingly valuable modality in diagnosing diseases of the gastrointestinal tract. The gradual compression technique and high-resolution multifrequency linear probes enable the displaying of changes in the intestinal wall [14]. Ultrasound plays an essential role in diagnosing diseases of the digestive tract, such as inflammatory bowel disease, small bowel obstruction, appendicitis, intussusception, and hypertrophic pyloric stenosis in newborns [15]. Factors that limit ultrasound examination of the abdominal organs, especially assessment of the digestive tract, are pain, pronounced flatulence, low spatial resolution, inability to display the rectum, and the distal part of the sigmoid colon. Recent studies, which compare Ultrasound and MRI in assessing the enlargement and inflammatory activity of Crohn's disease, indicate that ultrasound can localize the affected intestinal segments to some extent and the complications that accompany them [16, 17].

Sonographic lines of the intestinal wall correspond more to the interfaces than the wall's real histological layers. The central, thickened layer corresponds to the lamina submucosa, while the outer and inner hypoechoic layers correspond to the lamina mucosa and lamina muscularis respectively [18]. The wall is usually stratified if the lamina mucosa, submucosa, and muscularis propria are visible as separate layers. Loss of stratification is the inability to distinguish these layers or distinguish lamina mucosa from submucosa with visible muscularis.

The stomach wall's standard thickness is up to 5 mm, the small intestine up to 2 mm, and the large intestine up to 3 mm.

2.1.1.1 Examination technique and ultrasound findings

After the conventional abdominal ultrasound with a convex probe within the range of 2–5 MHz, the gastrointestinal tract examination is continued with high-frequency linear probes in the field of 5–10 MHz.

When inspecting the intestinal vortices, the gradual compression technique is used to expel air from the intestines.

Incompressibility and thickening are vital signs of a pathomorphological change of the wall. The intestine's pathomorphological altered segment is characterized by concentric wall thickening, absence or reduction of peristalsis, and lack of compressibility under pressure with an ultrasound probe [19] (**Figure 1**).

A wall thickness above 3 mm can be considered a pathological finding [20]. The discovery of a "pseudo-kidney" or "target sign" is the thickened, relatively hypoechoic intestinal wall surrounding the hyperechoic lumen, which is not specific and can be caused by other pathological conditions (neoplasms, intussusception, wall hematomas, hypertrophic pyloric ischemia, appendicitis, diverticulitis, etc.) [21]. A longitudinal view shows the tubular structure.

Some authors report a high percentage of detection of thickened intestinal convolutions (up to 90%) by high-resolution ultrasound, making it more challenging to determine the affected segment's exact length [22].

Therefore, the determination of the affected segment's length is estimated more reliably by other radiological methods [20].

An increasing number of authors emphasize the value of ultrasound in detecting and monitoring chronic inflammatory bowel disease, and in evaluating drug therapy

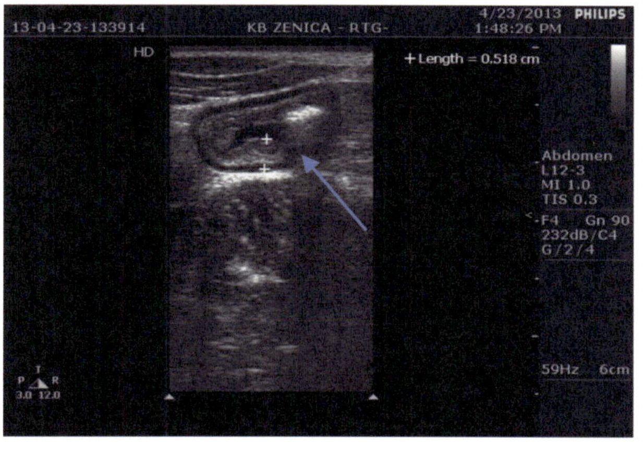

Figure 1.
Thickening of the terminal ileum wall.

effectiveness and presenting extramural complications (fistulas, abscesses, lymph nodes, free fluid) [23, 24] (**Figures 2** and **3**).

There are observations related to Crohn's disease that the loss of stratification due to wall edema correlates with the disease's active phase. In contrast, in the subacute and chronic phases, due to fibrosis, recognizable stratification from all five layers prevails [25].

2.1.2 CT enterography

It is a fast, non-invasive technique that uses a large amount of intestinal contrast material to better display the small intestine wall and lumen [26, 27].

CT enterography is not as sensitive as standard radiological methods in detecting mucosal damage. In comparison between them, it is superior in showing intramural and extraluminal changes [28] (**Figure 4**).

CT-proven mural thickening of the intestinal wall is the most crucial indicator of a pathological finding [29].

In the active inflammatory phase of the disease, contrast imbibition shows CT thickening of the wall and "stratification", which is indicated by a double halo - the "target sign" [29].

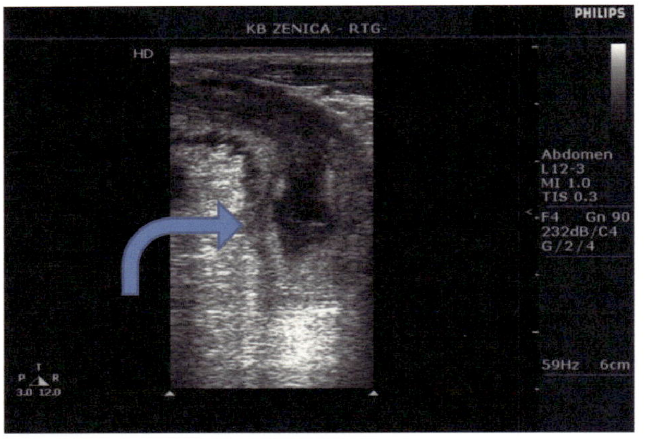

Figure 2.
Enterocutaneous fistula.

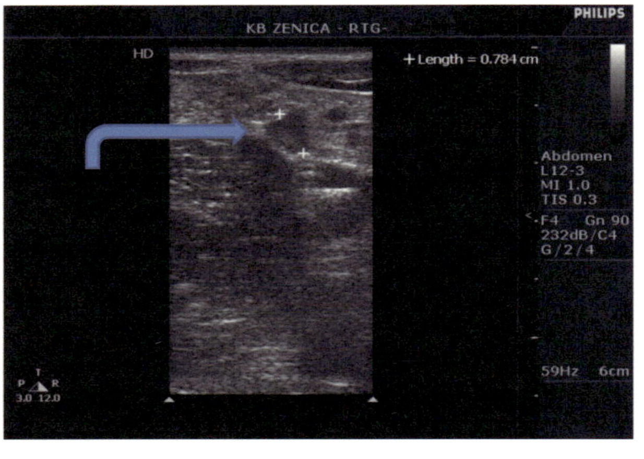

Figure 3.
Hypoechogenic, reactively altered lymph nodes.

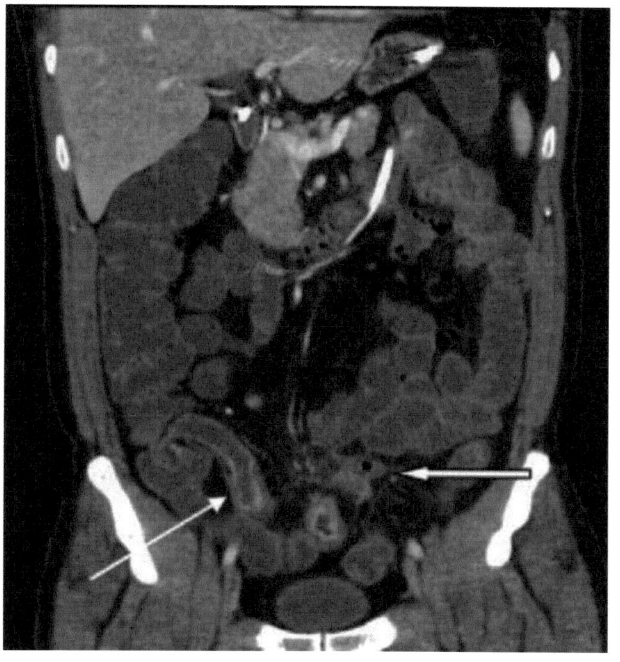

Figure 4.
CT enterography - thickening of the terminal ileum wall.

The main limiting factor in CT enterography is ionizing radiation, and it is unsuitable for the follow-up of patients with Crohn's disease.

2.1.3 Contrast MR enterography

Magnetic resonance imaging was introduced as an alternative method for detecting Crohn's disease and can be performed as MR enterography, or as MR enteroclysis [30–34].

MR enteroclysis is more demanding to perform and uncomfortable for the patient because it involves using a nasojejunal tube, and nowadays it is being avoided [35].

Technical advances with rapid sequences (GRE and EPI sequences, particularly HASTE) have minimized artifacts problem due to respiration and peristalsis [36]. Fat signal suppression is one of the technical modifications to better contrast the MR image [37].

The examination involves applying a more considerable amount of fluid orally to ensure the distension of the intestinal vortices, after which the MRI imaging itself is approached. Before the native and contrast sequences, an antispasmodic is administered intravenously to slow down the peristalsis and avoid bowel movement artifacts. After that, axial and coronal T1 and T2 sequences are recorded, as well as dynamic post-contrast recordings.

The fair spatial and temporal resolution of MR images, combined with a large amount of oral contrast agent that provides intestinal curvature distension, allows good visualization of the intestinal wall thickening, and edema thereof, which is useful for assessing Crohn's disease activity [38] (**Figure 5**).

A high signal in the T2 measured image as a well-known indicator of inflammation in human tissue should be a good indicator of inflammation in Crohn's disease.

The inflamed bowel wall in the T2-weighted image has a low-contrast resolution because the inflamed wall is more difficult to distinguish from the high signal of intraluminal fluid and perivisceral fatty tissue T2W sequence.

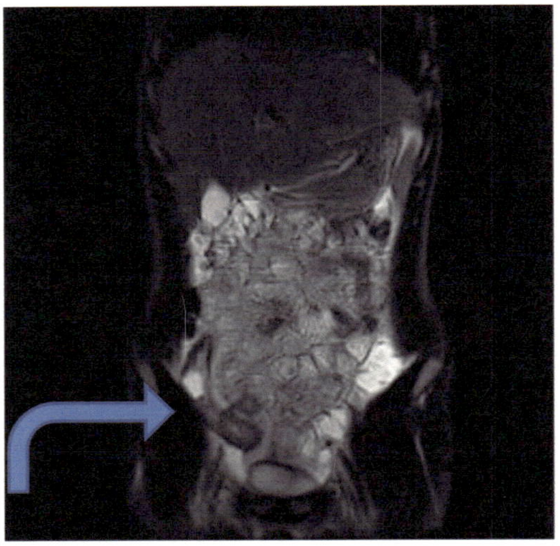

Figure 5.
T2 blade coronal mbh sequence: Distended intestinal loops with visible thickening of the terminal ileal wall.

Suppression of perivisceral adipose tissue signals with the "fat suppression" technique amplifies signal intensity of the inflamed intestine level. Also, superparamagnetic contrast (iron oxide particles) reduces the high intraluminal signal in the T2W-measured image.

Combining the above (fat suppression and superparamagnetic contrast) maximally improves the intestinal wall's high T2 signal. In other words, the mesenteric adipose tissue signal and the intraluminal content signal are "subtracted" from the display, which amplifies the inflamed intestinal wall signal in the T2W sequence.

Wall thickening, length of inflamed bowel and mural signal enhancement after intravenous administration of gadolinium correlate with Crohn's disease activity [39] (**Figure 6**).

MR enterography is easy to perform and has been proven to be useful for detecting active ileitis, assessing disease activity in the area of anastomoses, and identifying extraenteric complications [40–44] (**Figures 7–13**).

One of the earliest papers indicated a high sensitivity of over 90% in detecting fistulas in Crohn's disease [45].

The advantages of MRI imaging are:

- absence of ionizing radiation, which is especially crucial for the young population,
- possibility of using different parameters for the evaluation of inflammatory activity (T2 sequence),
- potential for making multiplanar and coronal representations,
- high signal intensity after the application of gadolinium in pathological changes of the intestinal wall,
- fair contrast resolution (display of wall edema) using fat suppression technique,
- high reliability to show fistulas.

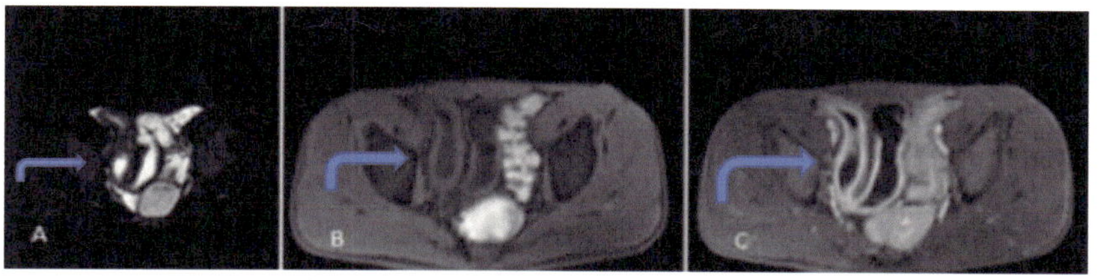

Figure 6.
(A) T2 blade fs axial multi breathe hold (mbh), (B) T1 vibe fs axial mbh, and (C) T1 vibe fs axial mbh postcontrast: Thickening of the ileal wall in Crohn's disease.

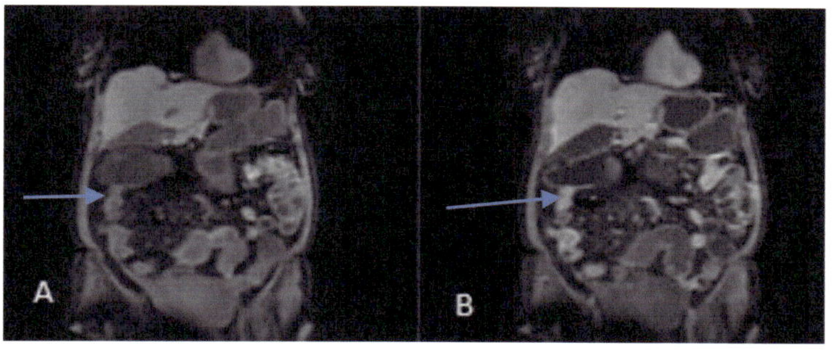

Figure 7.
(A) T1 vibe fs coronal mbh native and (B) T1 vibe fs coronal mbh after paramagnetic contrast agent application: Thickening of the ileal wall in the area of ileotransverso anastomosis.

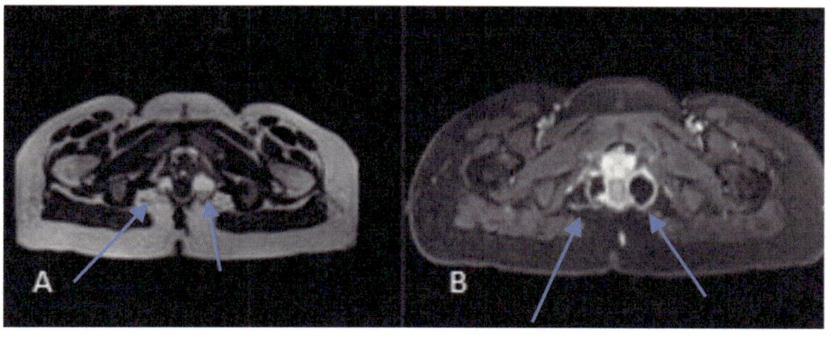

Figure 8.
(A) T2 blade transverse mbh and (B) T1 vibe transverse mbhpostcontrast: Perianal abscesses fused by retroanal fistula.

The disadvantages of MRI imaging are:

- high search price, and difficult availability,
- prolonged search time, and related claustrophobia,
- metal side of the body,
- lower spatial resolution.

2.1.4 Diffusion-weighted magnetic resonance imaging (DW MRI) and apparent diffusion coefficient (ADC)

Diffusion-weighted imaging (DWI) provides unique information about the observed tissue because the image contrast between different structures

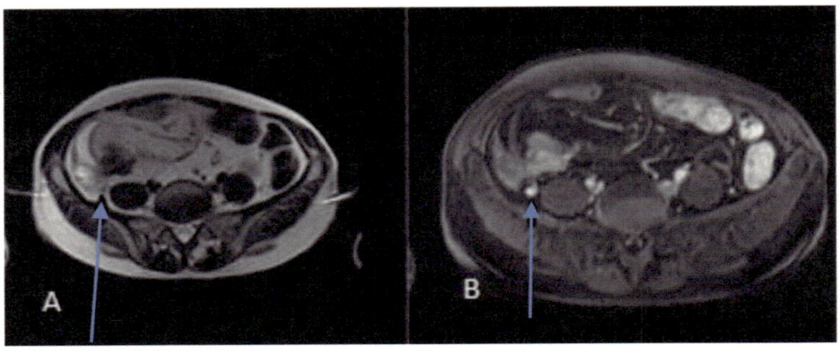

Figure 9.
(A) T2 blade transverse mbh and (B) T1 vibe transverse mbhpostcontrast: Significant lymph node along the Bauchini valve region.

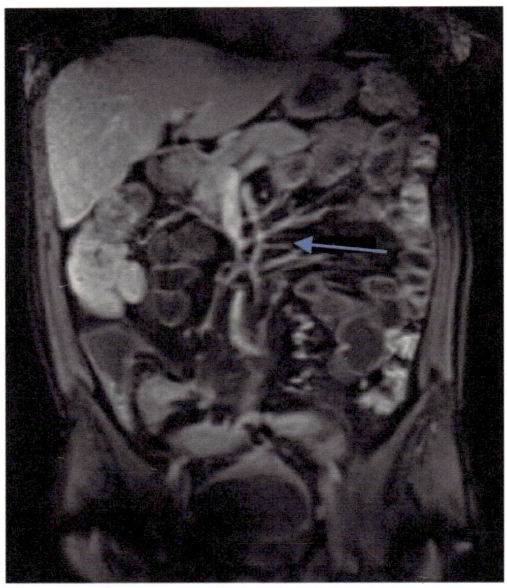

Figure 10.
T1 vibe coronal mbh postcontrast: Indicated blood vessels (vasa recta) as an indirect sign of inflammation.

in this technique depends on water molecules' local diffusion properties (**Figure 14**).

Diffusion-weighted imaging is a method by which we can accurately and non-invasively monitor proton diffusion of water molecules.

Diffusion is a physical term that describes the random movement of molecules without specific transport mechanisms [46].

Diffusion imaging of water is based on the natural sensitivity of MR signals to movement. In the presence of a magnetic field gradient, protons carried by water molecules' movement receive a phase shift of transverse magnetization.

Since other types of intravoxel incoherent movements, such as capillary perfusion, can produce effects similar to those of real diffusion, it has been proposed that the term ADC (Apparent Diffusion Coefficient) be used to quantify the results of in vivo diffusion imaging experiments.

The apparent diffusion coefficient (ADC) is calculated by comparing images with two or more different b-factor values allowing the diffusion to be quantified.

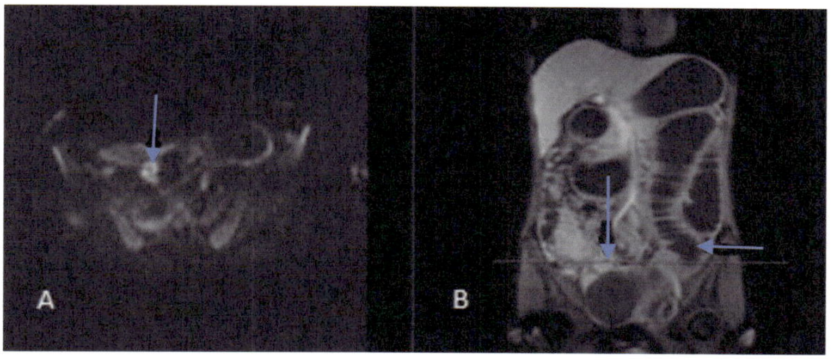

Figure 11.
(A) DWI and (B) T1 vibe fs coronal mbhpostcontrast sequence: Stenosis of the ileal segment with consequent distension of the proximal part of the small intestine - an indirect sign of affection.

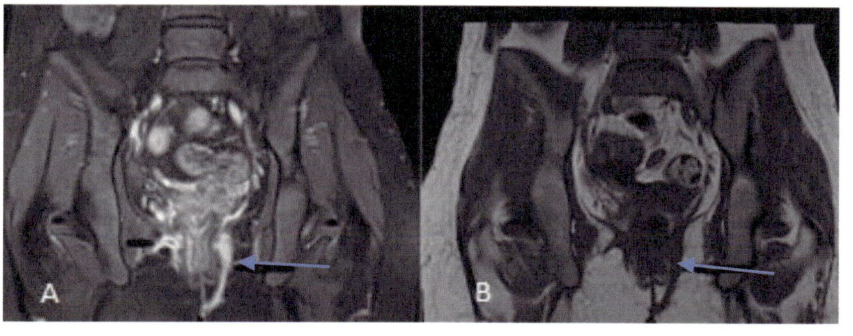

Figure 12.
(A) T1 vibe fs coronal mbh after and (B) pre-application of paramagnetic contrast agent (B): Perianal fistulas.

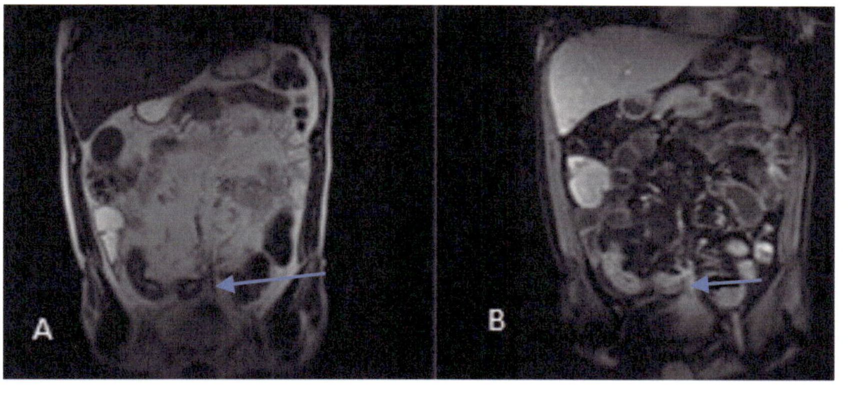

Figure 13.
(A) T2 blade coronal mbh and (B) T1 vibe fs coronal mbhpostcontrast: Enterovesical fistula.

Images in which the shade of the grayscale of an individual image element (pixel) is proportional to the apparent diffusion coefficient value are ADC maps.

Its high sensitivity limits clinical use of diffusion MR imaging to motion artifacts and limited hardware on conventional MR scanners.

The single-shot technique directly improves diffusion recording because it significantly reduces motion artifacts and increases the measured diffusion coefficient reliability by allowing many diffusion images to be obtained in a brief time interval. Thus, this technique is compatible with the clinical protocol [47].

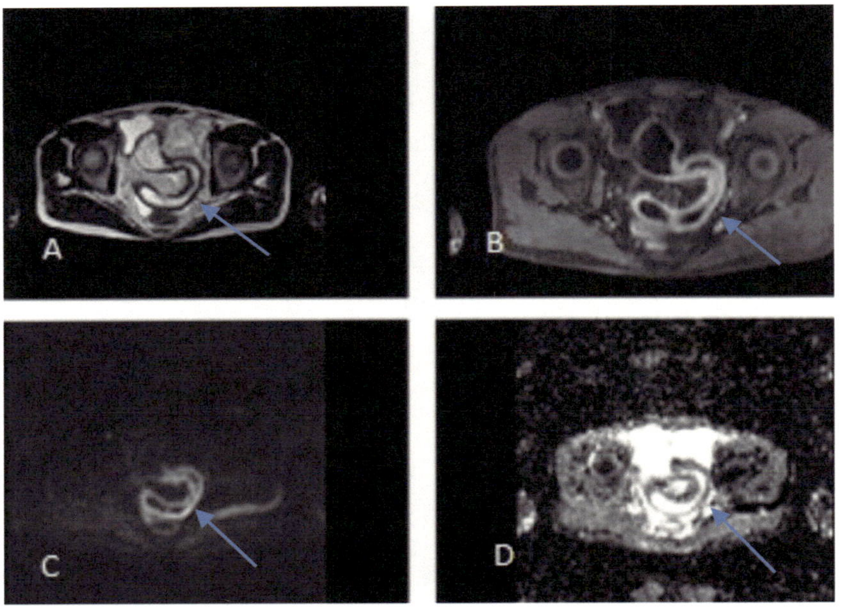

Figure 14.
(A) T2 blade transverse mbh, (B) T1 vibe fs transverse mbh, (C) DWI and (D) ADC map: Thickening of the ileal wall with visible free water diffusion restriction.

With this imaging technique, the whole signal from the tissue is canceled, so that only the signal of the molecules moving due to diffusion is displayed. The method is very demanding for the device, and only devices with good, strong, and fast gradients can cancel the signal enough not to see the "illumination of the T2 image", which can be sensed even with robust devices. These images are used daily to show the brain tissue that has experienced ischemia or stroke. Although the information obtained by diffusion measurements requires new studies, several reports have shown that diffusion imaging could become a powerful principle for the diagnosis of abdominal diseases [48–54].

3. What is the new gold standard?

Barium contrast tests and isotopes have been used to show inflammatory bowel disease, but they carry a risk of ionizing radiation exposure. Barium use is declining to result in fewer radiologists having the expertise and experience for such examinations - the lack of anatomical localizations limits isotopic studies.

CT is beneficial for assessing Crohn's disease complications, but it is burdened with high radiation.

CT enterography improves the visualization of the small bowel disease and allows the assessment of the disease activity.

Ultrasound has been increasingly used for the preliminary assessment of patients with potential IBD [55–59]. Although it is widely available and inexpensive, it depends on the experience of the doctor.

Finally, MRI is the most accurate tool for assessing the disease, its severity, and its prevalence [42–44, 60]. Pelvic MRI completely suppressed other techniques in the assessment of perianal fistulas [61].

According to the latest ECCO guidelines for the diagnosis of Crohn's disease, endoscopy and radiology are complementary techniques to define the site and extension of the disease so that optimal therapy can be planned [62].

4. Conclusions

Conventional ultrasound is a suitable orientation method in the initial evaluation of the patients with Crohn's disease. It can be used as an initial method for the patients who will subsequently undergo MRI enterography. CT is beneficial for assessing Crohn's disease complications, but it is burdened with high radiation.

Contrast MRI enterography provides an excellent assessment of disease activity, as well as the complications that accompany it. The method has a high sensitivity to changes seen in the patients with Crohn's disease; it offers detailed morphological and functional data on the small bowel disease and reliable evidence of normalcy; thus, it facilitates the final diagnosis of early or subtle structural abnormalities and helps to guide treatment and decisions on a further follow-up of patients. Contrast MRI enterography, in combination with DWI, is a comprehensive and safe method compared to reference - endoscopic examinations, and it should be considered as the preliminary examination for the detection of lesions in Crohn's disease, especially in children. Given the convenience and considering the safety and ease of the analysis, MRI enterography combined with DWI is suitable for repeated follow-up examinations, i.e. it can contribute to the follow-up of patients with Crohn's disease. Contrast MRI enterography combined with DWI is an excellent tool for evaluating complications of the underlying condition, especially for detecting fistulas, perianal fistulas in particular.

Conflict of interest

The authors declare no conflict of interest.

Author details

Bilal Imširović[1]*, Enver Zerem[2] and Emir Gušo[1]

1 Department of Radiology, General Hospital Sarajevo, Sarajevo, Bosnia and Herzegovina

2 Academy of Sciences and Arts of Bosnia and Herzegovina, Sarajevo, Bosnia and Herzegovina

*Address all correspondence to: bilal_imsirovic@yahoo.com

IntechOpen

© 2021 The Author(s). Licensee IntechOpen. This chapter is distributed under the terms of the Creative Commons Attribution License (http://creativecommons.org/licenses/by/3.0), which permits unrestricted use, distribution, and reproduction in any medium, provided the original work is properly cited.

References

[1] Loftus EV Jr. Clinical epidemiology of inflammatory bowel disease: Incidence, prevalence, and environmental influences. Gastroenterology. 2004;126:1504-1517.

[2] Mayberry JF, Judd D, Smart H, Rhodes J, Calcraft B, Morris JS. Crohn's disease in Jewishpeople - An epidemiological study in South-East Wales. 1986;35:237-240.

[3] Achitei D, Gologan E, Stefănescu G, Balan G. Clinical, biological and epidemiological aspects of inflammatory bowel diseases in North-East Romania. Rev Med ChirSoc Med Nat Iasi. 2013;117(1):16-22.

[4] Ng SC. Epidemiology of inflammatory bowel disease: focus on Asia. Best Pract Res ClinGastroenterol. 2014;28(3):363-372.

[5] Gore RM, Levine MS, Laufer I. Textbook ofgastroenterology. Philadelphia, Pa: Saunders 1994; 824-844.

[6] Gribajčević M, Nenad V, Mesihović R. Vodičzaupalnebolesticrijeva. Institutzanaučnoistraživački rad i razvoj KCUS. Sarajevo. 2007.

[7] Podolsky DK. Inflammatory bowel disease. Current Opinion in Gastroenterology 1995;11:289-291.

[8] Reeders JW. Inflammatory bowel disease. In: Radiologic-Pathologic Correlations. Eur Radiol 2000;10 (Suppl 2):S146–S156.

[9] Harb WJ.Crohn's Disease of the Colon, Rectum, and Anus. Surg Clin North Am. 2015;95(6):1195-1210.

[10] Lu KC, Hunt SR. Surgical management of Crohn's disease.Surg Clin North Am. 2013;93(1):167-185.

[11] Kilcoyne A, Kaplan JL, Gee MS. Inflammatory bowel disease imaging: Current practice and future directions. World J Gastroenterol. 2016;22(3):917-932.

[12] Zerem E. Comment on the article about the evaluation of transabdominal ultrasonography performed by a gastroenterologist in his office: why should not all clinicians use transabdominal ultrasonography on a routine basis? J Clin Gastroenterol. 2011;45(5): 476-477.

[13] Parente F, Greco S, Molteni M, Anderloni A, Sampietro GM, Danelli PG, Bianco R, Gallus S, Bianchi Porro G. Oral contrast enhanced bowel ultrasonography in the assessment of small intestine Crohn's disease. A prospective comparison with conventional ultrasound, x ray studies, and ileocolonoscopy. Gut. 2004;53:1652-1657.

[14] Brkljacic B. Dopler pri upalama u abdomenu. U: Brkljacic B. Dopler krvnih žila. Medicinska naklada, Zagreb. 2000;171-181.

[15] Derchi LE, Martinoli C, Valle M, Falchi M. Transabdominal ultrasound in the study of thegastrointestinal tract. In: Gandolfi L, Fukuda M. Current trends in digestive ultrasonography. FrontGastrointest Res. Karger, Basel. 1997;vol 24:56-78.

[16] Martínez MJ, Ripollés T, Paredes JM, Blanc E, Martí-Bonmatí L. Assessment of the extension and the inflammatory activity in Crohn's disease: comparison of ultrasound and MRI. Abdom Imaging. 2009;34:141-148.

[17] Schreyer GA, Menzel C, Friedrich C, Poschenrieder F, Egger L, Dornia C, Schill G, Dendl ML, Schacherer D, Girlich C,Jung ME. Comparison of high-resolution ultrasound and

MR-enterography in patients with inflammatory bowel disease. World J Gastroenterol. 2011;17(8): 1018-1025.

[18] Kimmey MB, Martin RW, Haggitt RC, Wang KY, Franklin DW, Silverstein FE.Histologic correlates of gastrointestinal ultrasound images. Gastroenterol 1989; 96:433-441.

[19] Barbaric-Babic V, Sjekavica I, Molnar M, Marinic J, Frkovic M, Dumic E, Krznaric Ž,Razumovic JJ. Sonography of Crohn's disease compared with barium study, CT andpatohistological examination. Eur Radiol (suppl.1) 2000;10:313.

[20] Barbaric-Babic V, Sjekavica I, Molnar M, Marinic J, Frkovic M, Krznaric Ž, Padovan ŠR. Crohn's disease-sonography,barium study,CT. Eur Radiol. 2001;11:C42.

[21] Limberg B. Diagnosis of chronic inflammatory bowel disease by ultrasonography. ZGastroenterol. 1999;37(6):495-508.

[22] Valette PJ, Rioux M, Pilleul F, Saurin JC, Fouque P, Henry L. Ultrasonography of chronic inflammatory bowel diseases. Eur Radiol. 2001;11(10):1859-1866.

[23] Andreas GS, Cynthia M, Chris F, Florian P, Lukas E, Christian D, Gabriela S, Lena MD, Doris S, Christl G, Ernst-Michael J. Comparison of high-resolution ultrasound and MR-enterography in patients with inflammatory bowel disease. World J Gastroenterol. 2011; 17(8):1018-1025.

[24] Dong J, Wang H, Zhao J, Zhu W, Zhang L, Gong J, Li Y, Gu L, Li J. Ultrasound as a diagnostic tool in detecting active Crohn's disease: a meta-analysis of prospective studies. EurRadiol. 2014;24(1):26-33.

[25] Tarjan Z, Toth G, Gyorke T, Mester A, Karlinger K, Mako EK. Ultrasound in Crohn'sdisease of the small bowel. Eur J Radiol. 2000;35(3):176-182.

[26] Grand DJ, Harris A, Loftus EV Jr. Imaging for luminal disease and complications: CT enterography, MR enterography, small-bowel follow-through, and ultrasound. Gastroenterol Clin North Am. 2012;41(2):497-512.

[27] Lim BK, Bux SI, Rahmat K, Lam SY, Liew YW. Evaluation of bowel distension and mural visualisation using neutral oralcontrast agents for multidetector-row computed tomography. Singapore Med J. 2012;53(11):732-736.

[28] Zhu QQ, Wang ZQ, Wu JT, Wang SA. Assessment of the diagnostic value of CT and X-ray enterography for small intestinal Crohn disease. Zhonghua Wei Chang WaiKeZaZhi. 2013;16(5):443-447.

[29] Amitai MM, Raviv-Zilka L, Hertz M, Erlich Z, Konen E, Ben-Horin S, Apter S. Main imaging features of Crohn's disease: Agreement between MR-enterography and CT-enterography. Isr Med Assoc J.2015;17(5):293-297.

[30] Kayhan A, Oommen J, Dahi F, Oto A. Magnetic resonance enterography in Crohn's disease: Standard and advanced techniques. World J Radiol. 2010;2(4):113-121.

[31] Kim YA. Role of computed tomography enterography/magnetic resonance enterography: Is it prime time?.ClinEndosc. 2010;45(3): 269-273.

[32] Oommen J, Oto A. Contrast-enhancedMRI of the small bowel in Crohn's disease. AbdomImaging. 2011;6(2):134-141.

[33] Ziech ML, Bossuyt PM, Laghi A, Lauenstein TC, Taylor SA, Stoker J. Grading luminal Crohn's disease: which

MRI features are considered as important?Eur J Radiol. 2012;81(4): e467-72.

[34] Florie J, Wasser MN, Arts-Cieslik K, Akkerman EM, Siersema PD, Stoker J. Dynamic contrast-enhanced MRI of the bowel wall for assessment of disease activity in Crohn's disease. AJR Am J Roentgenol. 2006;186:1384-1392.

[35] Gee MS, Harisinghani MG. MRI in patients with inflammatory bowel disease. J MagnReson Imaging. 2011;33(3):527-534.

[36] Papanikolaou N, Grammatikakis J, Maris TG, Chrysou E, Prassopoulos P, Gourtsoyiannis N. A comprehensive MRI protocol for small bowel studies. Eur Radiol 2001;11:C15.

[37] Štern-Padovan R. CT i MR u gastroeneterologiji. U: Vucelic B. i suradnici.Gastroenterologija i hepatologija. Medicinska naklada, Zagreb. 2002; 327-338.

[38] Tolan DJ, Greenhalgh R, Zealley IA, Halligan S, Taylor SA. MR enterographic manifestations of small bowel Crohn disease. Radiographics. 2010;30: 367-384.

[39] Shoenut JP, Semelka RC, Silverman R, Yaffe CS, Micflikier AB. Magnetic resonance imaging in inflammatory bowel disease. J Clin Gastroenterol. 1993;17:73-78.

[40] Li W, Yuan F, Zhou Z. Imaging diagnosis of perianal fistula in Crohn disease. Zhonghua Wei Chang WaiKeZaZhi. 2014;17(3):215-218.

[41] Costa-Silva L, Brandão AC. MR enterography for the assessment of small bowel diseases. MagnReson Imaging Clin N Am. 2013;21(2): 365-383.

[42] Nieun S, Seong HP, Kyung JK, Bo KK, Yedaun L, Suk KY et al. MR Enterography for the evaluation of small-bowel inflammation in Crohn disease by using diffusion-weighted imaging without intravenous contrast material: a prospective noninferiority study. Radiology. 2016;278(3):762-772.

[43] Aysegul C, Suleyman B, Sukru O, Eser B, Sami F. Can diffusion weighted imaging be used as an alternative to contrast-enhanced imaging on magnetic resonance enterography for the assessment of active inflammation in Crohn disease? Medicine (Baltimore). 2020;99(8):e19202.

[44] Gabriele M, Chiara DV, Marina A, Marianna G, Ronerta C, Gaia C, Vittorio M, Roberto G. Detection of Crohn's disease with diffusion images versus contrast-enhanced images in pediatric using MR enterography with histopathological correlation. Radiol Med. 2019;124(12):1306-1314.

[45] Koelbel G, Schmiedl U, Majer MC,et al. diagnosis of fistulae and sinus tracts in patientswith Crohn's disease: value of MR imaging. AM J Roentgenol. 1989;152:999-1003.

[46] Agutter PS, Malone PC, Wheatley DN. Diffusion theory in biology: A relic ofmechanistic materialism. J Hist Biol. 2000; 33:71-111.

[47] Baltić i saradnici. Nuklearnamagnetnarezonancija u onkologiji. Znamenje, Novi Sad. 2002.

[48] Mentzel HJ, Reinsch S, Kurzai M, Stenzel M. Magnetic resonance imaging in children and adolescents with chronic inflammatory bowel disease. World J Gastroenterol. 2014;20(5):1180-1191.

[49] Tajima T, Akahane M, Takao H, Akai H, Kiryu S, Imamura H, Watanabe Y, Kokudo N, Ohtomo K. Detection of liver metastasis: is diffusion-weighted imaging needed in Gd-EOB-DTPA-enhanced MR imaging for evaluation of colorectal

liver metastases?Jpn J Radiol. 2012;30(8):648-58.

[50] Matsuki M, Inada Y, Nakai G, et al. Diffusion-weighed MR imaging of pancreatic carcinoma. Abdom Imaging. 2007;32:481-483.

[51] Zhang J, Tehrani YM, Wang L, Ishill NM, Schwartz LH, Hricak H. Renal masses: characterization with diffusion-weighted MR imaging—a preliminary experience. Radiology. 2008;247:458-464.

[52] Koh DM, Sohaib A. Diffusion-weighted imaging of the male pelvis.RadiolClin North Am. 2012;50(6):1127-44.

[53] Leufkens AM, Kwee TC, van den Bosch MA, Mali WP, Takahara T, Siersema PD. Diffusion-weighted MRI for the detection of colorectal polyps: feasibility study.MagnResonImaging. 2013;31(1):28-35.

[54] Hosonuma T, Tozaki M, Ichiba N, et al. Clinical usefulness of diffusion-weighted imaging using low and high b-values to detect rectal cancer. MagnReson Med Sci. 2006;5:173-177.

[55] Clara BC, Mariangela G, Daniele G, Dario C, Mirella F. Role of bowel ultrasound in the diagnosis and follow-up of patients with Crohn's disease. Ultrasound Med Biol. 2017;43(4):725-734.

[56] Rosa C, Helena R, Giovanni M. Bowel thickening in Crohn's disease: fibrosis or inflammation? Diagnostic ultrasound imaging tools. Inflamm Bowel Dis. 2017;23(1):23-34.

[57] Kerri N, Christian M, Rune W, Giovanni M. Diagnostic accuracy of MRE and ultrasound for Crohn's disease. Lancet GastroenterolHepatol. 2019;4(2):95-96.

[58] Kumar S, Hakim A, Alexakis C, Chhaya V, Tzias D, Pilcher J, Vlahos J, Pollok R. Small intestinal contrast ultrasonography for the detection of small bowel complications in Crohn's disease: Correlation with intraoperative findings and magnetic resonance enterography. J GastroenterolHepatol. 2015 Jan;30(1):86-91.

[59] Imsirovic B, Zerem E, Guso E, Djedovic M, Cengic A, Baljic R, Merhemic Z, Efendic A. Comparison of conventional ultrasound and contrast enhanced magnetic resonance (MR) enterography in evaluation patients with Crohn's disease. Acta Inform Med. 2018;26(2.000): 93-97.

[60] Imširović B, Zerem E, Efendić A, Mekić AA, Zerem O, Djedović M. Significance of diffusion weighted imaging (DWI) as an improving factor in contrast enhanced magnetic resonance imaging (MRI) enterography in evaluation of patients with Crohn's disease. Med Glas. 2018;15(2):145-151.

[61] Dambha F, Tanner J, Carroll N. Diagnostic imaging in Crohn's disease: what is the new gold standard? Best Pract Res ClinGastroenterol. 2014 Jun;28(3):421-436.

[62] Fernando G, Axel D, Vito A, Herbert T, Gert VA, James OL et al. 3rd European evidence-based consensus on the diagnosis and management of Crohn's disease 2016: Part 1: Diagnosis and medical management. Journal of Crohn's and Colitis. 2017:3-25.

Section 3

Inflammatory Bowel Disease

Chapter 3

Endoscopy in Small Bowel Crohn's Disease

Isabel Garrido, Susana Lopes and Guilherme Macedo

Abstract

Crohn's disease (CD) is a complex disorder with variable age of onset, disease location and behavior. It is characterized by a transmural inflammation that may involve any portion of the gastrointestinal tract. Ileocolonoscopy with biopsy is established as the first-line investigation for suspected CD. However, small bowel involvement is more difficult to assess by conventional endoscopy. Therefore, radiological imaging should also be performed to complement ileocolonoscopy in all patients with suspected CD. Recently, video capsule endoscopy and device-assisted enteroscopy have revolutionized the management of small bowel CD. In fact, video capsule endoscopy is a non-invasive test that provides the visualization of the entire small bowel mucosa, which can assist in the diagnosis of CD and assess the therapeutic response. On the other hand, device-assisted enteroscopy enables direct tissue sampling for histopathology confirmation when traditional endoscopy, video capsule endoscopy and cross-sectional imaging are inconclusive. Moreover, it allows therapeutic interventions such as balloon stricture dilation. In this chapter, we review the role of endoscopy in the diagnosis and management of patients with small bowel CD.

Keywords: Inflammatory bowel disease, Crohn's disease, endoscopy, small bowel

1. Introduction

Crohn's disease (CD) is an idiopathic inflammatory disorder with genetic, immunologic and environmental influences [1]. It is characterized by a transmural inflammation that may involve any portion of the luminal gastrointestinal tract, from the oral cavity to the perianal area. The diagnosis is based on the combination of clinical, biochemical, radiological, endoscopic and histological findings. CD is a chronic and progressive disease, marked by frequent relapses which usually require repeated investigations.

The most common symptoms of CD are diarrhea, abdominal pain and fatigue. However, clinical manifestations can be very heterogeneous, depending on the disease location and phenotype. Patients with CD often show laboratory evidence of inflammatory activity and anemia. In addition, fecal calprotectin and serum C-reactive protein are useful markers to detect and monitor inflammation. The endoscopic hallmark of CD is the patchy distribution of inflammation and mucosal biopsies usually show focal inflammation (rather than diffuse), crypt distortion and/or granulomas. Finally, cross-sectional imaging techniques provide information about the bowel wall and extra-enteric soft tissues and, therefore, can better classify disease phenotype and behavior.

Endoscopy has major implications not only for the diagnosis of CD but also for treatment and follow-up. Indeed, ileocolonoscopy and upper gastrointestinal endoscopy have well-established roles in assessing disease activity and therapeutic intervention. However, the small bowel is one of the most common areas affected in patients with CD, which is often inaccessible to conventional endoscopy. In addition, at the time of diagnosis, up to 30% of patients have only small bowel involvement, especially in the young ones [2, 3]. The advent of video capsule endoscopy and both balloon-assisted and spiral enteroscopy is revolutionizing the management of small bowel CD [4]. In fact, these techniques allowed direct visualization of the entire small bowel which can assist in the diagnosis of CD. Moreover, device-assisted enteroscopy enables direct tissue sampling and allows therapeutic interventions. In this chapter, we aim to review the role of small bowel endoscopy in the management of patients with CD.

2. Diagnosis

2.1 Ileocolonoscopy

Colonoscopy with intubation of the terminal ileum and multiple biopsies is recommended as part of the initial evaluation of patients with suspected CD [5]. It has been reported a successful ileal intubation rate as high as % when the cecum is reached [6]. A minimum of two biopsies from five different sites, including the rectum and the ileum, should be obtained for a reliable diagnosis of CD. Samples are preferably obtained both from areas which are involved by the disease and from uninvolved areas. Mucosal changes suggestive of CD include discontinuous segments of edema, friability, ulcerations, fistulous orifices and stenosis (**Figure 1**). With respect to the histological exam, macroscopic and microscopic features include discontinuous chronic inflammation, with lymphocytes and plasma cells, focal crypt distortion and granulomas. Although the presence of granulomatous inflammation is helpful, it is not required for diagnosis and is seen in only 33% of patients with CD [7].

Ileocolonoscopy is also helpful for the detection of stenosis, allowing tissue sampling for pathological diagnosis of dysplasia and cancer. Complementary radiological techniques to rule out additional stenotic lesions are necessary when the lesion is impassable with the endoscope.

Attempts to quantify the distribution and severity of mucosal involvement of the colon and the ileum in patients with CD have led to the development of multiple endoscopic scoring systems. Endoscopic scores that have been validated for ileocolonoscopy include both the Crohn's Disease Endoscopic Index of Severity (CDEIS) [8]

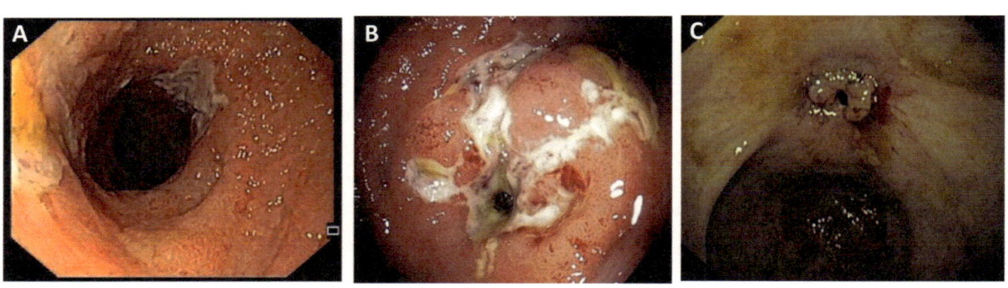

Figure 1.
Endoscopic appearance of Crohn's disease - discontinuous segments of edema, friability, ulcerations (A) and stenosis (B and C).

and the Simple Endoscopic Score for Crohn's Disease (SES-CD) [9]. The CDEIS includes six endoscopic variables (presence of deep ulcers, superficial ulcers, nonulcerated stenosis, ulcerated stenosis, proportion of ulcerated surface and proportion of surface affected by disease), assessed in five bowel segments (terminal ileum, right colon, transverse, left colon and sigmoid, rectum) (**Table 1**). The CDEIS is complicated to use and requires training and experience. Therefore, it is used mainly in clinical trials. On the other hand, the SES-CD has been helpful to translate endoscopic activity into clinically meaningful and is easier to use and understand. The SES-CD includes four variables, each considered in five bowel segments (ulcer size, extent of ulcerated surface, extent of affected surface and stenosis) (**Table 2**).

	Ileum	**Right colon**	**Transverse colon**	**Left colon**	**Rectum**	**Sum**	
Deep ulceration (0 for none, 12 points if present)							Total 1
Superficial ulceration (0 for none, 6 points if present)							Total 2
Surface involved by disease (cm)							Total 3
Surface involved by ulceration (cm)							Total 4
Total 1 + 2 + 3 + 4							Total A
Number of segments totally or partially explored							n
Total A divided by n							Total B
Quote 3 if ulcerated stenosis anywhere							C
Quote 3 if nonulcerated stenosis anywhere							D
Total B + C + D							CDEIS

Table 1.
Crohn's disease endoscopic index of severity (CDEIS). CDEIS includes deep ulceration (no = 0, yes = 12), superficial ulceration (no = 0, yes = 6), surface involved by disease (0–10), ulcerated surface (0–10), and ulcerated or non-ulcerated stenosis (no = 0, yes = 3), each considered in five ileocolonic segments. Severe disease: CDEIS ≥12, moderate disease: CDEIS = 9–12, mild disease: CDEIS = 3–9, remission: CDEIS <3.

Variable	**0**	**1**	**2**	**3**
Size of ulcers	None	Aphthous ulcers (0.2–0.5 cm)	Large ulcers (0.5-2 cm)	Very large ulcers (>2 cm)
Ulcerated surface	None	<10%	10–30%	>30%
Affected surface	None	<50%	50–75%	>75%
Presence of narrowing	None	Single, can be passed	Multiple, can be passed	Impassible

Table 2.
Simple endoscopic score for Crohn's disease (SES-CD). SES-CD = sum of all variables of each explored segment (ileum, right colon, transverse colon, left colon and rectum). Severe disease: SES-CD ≥16, moderate disease: SES-CD = 7–15, mild disease: SES-CD = 3–6, inactive disease: SES-CD <3.

It is important to note that up to 25% of patients have isolated proximal small bowel disease beyond the reach of even complete ileocolonoscopy [10]. Therefore, radiological imaging should be performed in all patients with suspected CD to complement ileocolonoscopy.

2.2 Upper gastrointestinal endoscopy

The presence of CD of the upper gastrointestinal tract, including the duodenum, is uncommon in adults, with most studies showing a prevalence range of 0.3–5% [11]. Moreover, the majority of patients are asymptomatic at the time of evaluation [12]. However, it is important to note that CD in the proximal gastrointestinal tract is associated with a worse prognosis and there is usually a low threshold to initiate therapy with anti-tumor necrosis factor (TNF).

CD involving the upper gastrointestinal tract is almost invariably accompanied by small or large bowel involvement [13]. Esophagogastroduodenoscopy is recommended in patients with upper gastrointestinal signs and symptoms, being still debated whether asymptomatic adult CD patients should routinely undergo upper endoscopy [6]. In fact, esophagogastroduodenoscopy may support the diagnosis when it is difficult to obtain a histological diagnosis of CD. In addition, a more recent prospective registry reported a higher prevalence of upper gastrointestinal involvement in asymptomatic patients than initially expected, suggesting a place for a standard gastroscopy to correctly evaluate disease extent at diagnosis [12].

Endoscopic features suggestive of upper gastrointestinal involvement include mucosal nodularity, aphthous ulcers, superficial erosions, antral thickening and duodenal strictures [1]. Histologic changes consistent with CD are granulomatous inflammation, focally enhanced gastritis and focal cryptitis of the duodenum.

In the presence of upper tract stenosis, balloon dilatation is recommended as first-line therapy, followed by proton pump inhibitors as second-line and steroids/thiopurines/surgery as third-line [14]. Currently, there is no credible evidence to support the best modality to assess response to treatment of upper gastrointestinal CD, therefore it must be primarily monitored by the reference standard endoscopy.

2.3 Video capsule endoscopy

Video capsule endoscopy is a method of endoluminal examination of the small bowel using a wireless capsule-shaped tool which is swallowed and then propelled through the gastrointestinal tract by gut motility [15]. Preparations for a video capsule endoscopy study usually include 8–12 hours' fasting and some method of bowel cleansing (e.g. polyethylene glycol preparation). During the battery life of the capsule, images of the small bowel are recorded and reformatted into a continuous video file. After 8–10 hours, the antenna and storage unit are removed and the images transferred to a computer with specially adapted software. Images are then downloaded, processed and examined by a trained gastroenterologist (**Figure 2**).

In addition to the small-bowel capsule, there are currently two more: the esophageal and the colon capsules [16]. The esophageal capsule is the same size as the small bowel capsule, but has lenses on both ends of the 'pill.' The capsule battery life is only 20 minutes (vs. 8–12 hours for small-bowel capsules), cameras are located on both ends of the capsule and take 18 frames per second (vs. 2–3 frames per second for small-bowel capsules). On the other hand, the second-generation colon capsule endoscope is equipped with two high-resolution cameras providing a viewing angle of 172° in front and back, senses the moving speed of the capsule endoscope and captures 4 to 35 images per second [17]. This capsule was primarily utilized

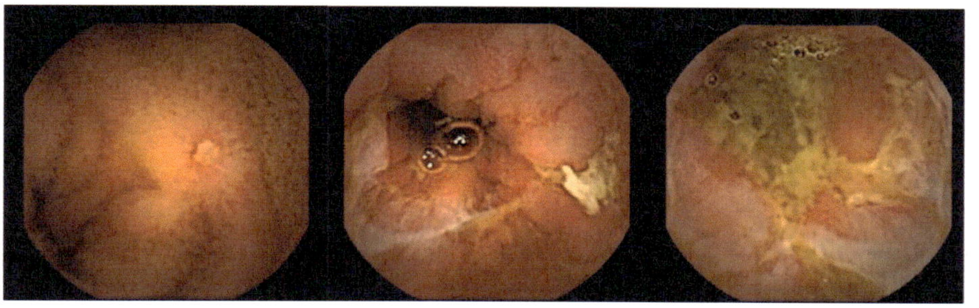

Figure 2.
Video capsule endoscopy images showing mucosal inflammation and ulcerations consistent with a diagnosis of Crohn's disease.

in screening for colonic neoplasia, particularly in situations such as incomplete colonoscopy. However, it can play a key role in the diagnosis and evaluation of CD extent, severity and prognosis, with treatment modifications based on data from capsule examination.

Video capsule endoscopy is a useful adjunct in the diagnosis of patients with small bowel CD since it allows for direct visualization of the mucosa of the entire small intestine. It is able to identify mucosal lesions compatible with CD in patients in whom conventional endoscopic and small bowel radiographic imaging modalities have been nondiagnostic, especially in the proximal small bowel [18]. Several meta-analyses have examined the diagnostic yield of video capsule endoscopy in the evaluation of patients with suspected CD and showed that it is superior to small bowel barium studies, computed tomography enterography and ileocolonoscopy, with an incremental yield of diagnosis of 32%, 47% and 22%, respectively [19]. Moreover, video capsule endoscopy has a negative predictive value of 96%, essentially ruling out small bowel CD [20]. On the other hand, a study examining the sensitivity and specificity of different endoscopic and radiologic exams showed that the specificity of video capsule endoscopy was significantly lower than the other tests [21]. In fact, detected lesions are nonspecific and cannot be distinguished from those seen in patients treated by nonsteroidal anti-inflammatory drugs (NSAIDs). Therefore, video capsule endoscopy should be reserved for cases in which ileocolonoscopy plus small bowel radiography is not diagnostic, but there is a high rate of CD suspicion.

Although there are no validated diagnostic criteria for the diagnosis of CD, the presence of more than three small bowel ulcerations, in the absence of NSAIDs ingestion for at least 1 month before the exam, constitutes the most commonly used diagnostic criterion in practice [22]. In addition, there are currently two validated indexes available, the Capsule Endoscopy Crohn's Disease Activity Index (CECDAI) [23] and the Lewis Score [24], which assess the disease location and activity of small bowel involvement. The CECDAI was validated in a multicenter prospective study of patients with isolated small bowel CD and evaluates the following three endoscopic parameters: inflammation, extent of disease and strictures for both the proximal and the distal segments of the small bowel, based on the transit time of the capsule (**Table 3**). The Lewis score is another scoring system based on the evaluation of three endoscopic parameters: villous appearance, ulcers and strictures (**Table 4**). The small bowel is divided into three equal parts and, for each tertile, a subscore is determined. The Lewis Score is the sum of the worst affected tertile plus the stenosis score. Both the scoring systems are incorporated into the software platform of the capsules and assists in the quantification of small bowel inflammatory burden and diagnosis of CD.

Parameter	Score and descriptor
A - Inflammation	0 - None 1 – Mild to moderate (edema, hyperemia or denudation) 2 – Severe (edema, hyperemia or denudation) 3 – Bleeding, exudate, erosion aphthae, ulcers <0.5 cm 4 – Pseudopolyp, ulcers 0.5-2 cm 5 – Ulcers >2 cm
B – Extent of disease	0 – None 1 – Sigle segment (focal disease) 2–2-3 segments (patchy disease) 3 - >3 segments (diffuse disease)
C - Stricture	0 – None 1 – Single-passed 2 – Multiple-passed 3 – Obstruction (non-passage)

Table 3.
Capsule endoscopy Crohn's disease activity index (CECDAI). CECDAI = proximal segment (A x B + C) + distal segment (A x B+C). Clinical or endoscopic remission: CEDAI <4.

Parameter	Descriptor or number	Longitudinal extent	Descriptor
Villous appearance	0- Normal 1- Edematous	8- Short-segment (<10%) 12- Long-segment (11–50%) 20- Whole tertile (>50%)	1- Single 14- Patchy 17- Diffuse
Ulcers	0- Normal 3- Single 5- Few (2–7) 10- Multiple (≥8)	5- Short-segment (<10%) 10- Long-segment (11–50%) 15- Whole tertile (>50%)	9- < ¼ 12- ¼ - ½ 18- > ½
Stenosis	0- None 14- Single 20- Multiple	2- Nonulcerated 24- Ulcerated	7- Transversed 10- Not transversed

Table 4.
Lewis score. Score total = worst-affected tertile villous appearance and ulcers plus stenosis score. Clinically insignificant inflammation: Lewis score <135, mild inflammation: Lewis score = 135–790, moderate to severe inflammation: Lewis score >790.

Video capsule endoscopy may also identify a site for directed visualization with other endoscopic techniques. In fact, it can be complementary to device-assisted endoscopy since findings may help direct the most effective route of intubation (oral versus anal), in order to obtain a histopathological diagnosis or therapeutic intervention.

In addition, video capsule endoscopy allows detection of subtle small bowel lesions, which may affect the therapeutic management. Because of the high sensitivity of video capsule endoscopy, it has a potential role in the assessment of mucosal healing after drug therapy and can be used in the follow-up of treated patients. In fact, video capsule endoscopy has a significant impact on disease management and is associated with earlier escalation of therapy. In the largest retrospective series of patients with established CD that were evaluated with video capsule endoscopy, a change in management was suggested in 40–52% of individuals [25, 26].

The main advantage of video capsule endoscopy is the ability to visualize all of the small bowel with minimal discomfort for the patient. However, it lacks therapeutic capabilities and there is some risk of impaction due to possible strictures.

The capsule retention rate in patients with suspected CD is 1.5–5.4% but can reach 13% in those with established CD, particularly if there are known intestinal stenosis [27, 28]. Therefore, those with obstructive symptoms or established CD of the small bowel should always have small bowel imaging and/or patency capsule evaluation before video capsule endoscopy to decrease the risk of capsule retention. Video capsule endoscopy is considered safe if the patency capsule is excreted before 30 hours, an intact capsule is excreted after 30 hours or passage to the colon of an intact patency capsule has been radiologically confirmed. Another disadvantage of video capsule endoscopy is that the quality of images is not comparable to the view achieved at conventional endoscopy with gas insufflation. In addition, it has been reported that the caecum is not reached in 8–40% of video capsule endoscopy studies [22, 29]. Finally, the most serious complication reported with video capsule endoscopy is perforation, which has been exceedingly rare [30].

2.4 Device-assisted endoscopy

Device-assisted endoscopy is a generic term for any endoscopic technique that includes assisted progression (i.e. balloons and overtubes) and comprises double-balloon enteroscopy, single-balloon enteroscopy and spiral enteroscopy [31]. Device-assisted endoscopy allows direct mucosal visualization of the entire small bowel as well as tissue sampling and therapeutic intervention (**Figure 3**). However, it is technically challenging and may require a bi-directional approach, deep sedation or general anesthesia.

Double-balloon enteroscopy was introduced in 2001 as the first method for device-assisted enteroscopy [32]. It allows deep intubation of the small bowel by pleating the bowel onto a long and flexible endoscope fitted with an overtube. The endoscope and the accompanying overtube have balloons at their distal end. By intermittent inflation and deflation of these two balloons, combined with instrument insertion and retraction, large portions of the small bowel can be visualized directly. Oral and anal routes are used to achieve a complete small bowel examination.

Single-balloon enteroscopy is able to achieve a complete examination of the small bowel using principles similar to double-balloon enteroscopy. However, in contrast to double-balloon enteroscopy, this exam has only one balloon at the distal end of the overtube, which simplifies the preparation of the scope before starting the procedure. Single-balloon enteroscopy uses scope tip angulation and suction instead of balloon inflation to maintain a stable position while advancing the overtube.

Spiral enteroscopy is based on a completely different concept, by pleating of the bowel on the instrumentation shaft by active rotation instead of applying pushing force. The distal end of the overtube harbors a flexible spiral thread for pleating the small intestine over the overtube. By manually rotating the overtube, the spiral engages the small bowel which is thus pleated onto or unpleated from the overtube, respectively, depending on the direction of the spiral rotation. Spiral assisted endoscopy has been approved for both anterograde and retrograde enteroscopy.

The Motorized Spiral Enteroscope is a new technology with an incorporated user-controlled motor contained in the handle of the endoscope [33]. This would offer the possibility to accelerate the procedure, facilitate insertion and simplify the technique with a single operator. Recently, Beyna et al. demonstrated that the Motorized Spiral Enteroscope is effective for diagnostic and therapeutic antegrade enteroscopy and may compare favorably with traditional methods of deep enteroscopy in ease of use and procedural duration [34].

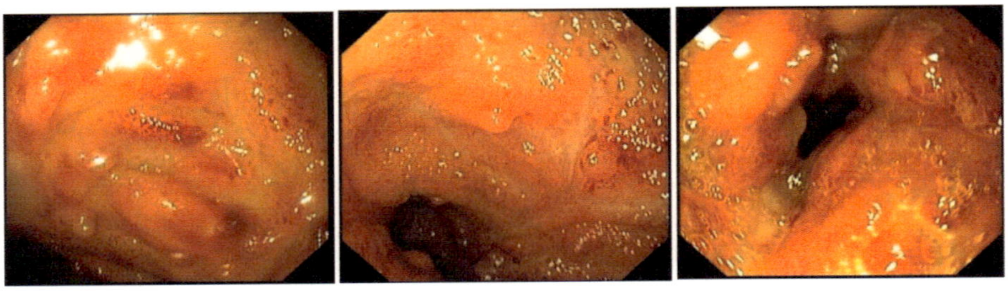

Figure 3.
Device-assisted endoscopy images showing mucosal inflammation and ulcerations consistent with a diagnosis of Crohn's disease.

Device-assisted endoscopy is not part of routine diagnostic testing in patients with suspected CD and should not be the first-line procedure in the evaluation of small bowel [1]. However, it may provide additional information when it is required biopsy of small bowel tissue to histological corroboration. Indeed, compared with video capsule endoscopy and small bowel imaging techniques, the advantages of device-assisted endoscopy include the evaluation of atypical lesions, the ability to obtain biopsies for histopathology and the potential for therapeutic intervention.

Device-assisted endoscopy studies in individuals with suspected CD have not included large numbers of patients but report a diagnostic yield as high as 80% [35]. In fact, device-assisted endoscopy is more sensitive in detecting lesions in patients with suspected CD than multiple radiographic imaging techniques. Nevertheless, because of the invasive and potentially time-consuming nature of the exam, it should be reserved for patients with high clinical suspicion of CD despite negative conventional studies (including ileocolonoscopy, video capsule endoscopy and radiographic imaging), particularly if endoscopic and histologic finding would alter disease management or potential therapeutic intervention is required [36]. In a prospective trial, positive findings at device-assisted enteroscopy led to a step-up of medical therapy in 74% of patients, leading to clinical remission in 88% [37]. In addition, device-assisted endoscopy may be preferable to video capsule endoscopy if there is a clinical suspicion of obstruction because it may allow therapeutic intervention and be safer, simply by avoiding capsule retention.

In patients with established CD, device-assisted endoscopy is indicated when endoscopic visualization and biopsies are necessary from areas of the small bowel inaccessible to conventional endoscopy [1]. Usually, previous video capsule endoscopy provides information on the optimal route of approach (oral or rectal) and lesion location. Adhesions may limit examination by device-assisted endoscopy and, in these circumstances, double-balloon enteroscopy may be preferred to single-balloon enteroscopy. In addition, device-assisted endoscopy has the capacity for endoscopic therapy, including dilation of small bowel strictures, removal of impacted capsules and treatment of bleeding lesions (*vide infra*).

Overall, diagnostic device-assisted endoscopy is safe, with few reports of complications (<1%) [38]. However, there appears to be an increased risk of complications in the case of active CD or previous intestinal surgery. The risk of perforation is 0.12% without therapeutic intervention and 1.74% with therapeutic intervention, the majority of which occurred after stricture dilatation [39]. Bleeding occurs in approximately 2.5%. In addition, device-assisted endoscopy involves risks related to sedation, in contrast to video capsule endoscopy where no sedation is required.

3. Treatment

3.1 Treatment of intestinal strictures

Strictures in CD develop during the course of the disease or as the presenting feature and are believed to result from partial healing and localized fibrosis. In addition, almost one-third of CD patients develop an anastomotic stricture after ileocecal resection/right hemicolectomy [40]. As a progressive disease, anastomotic strictures will be more likely over time.

Immunomodulators and biologic agents have been widely used for the treatment of CD, however endoscopic dilatation is a preferred technique for the management of symptomatic and mild to moderate stenosing disease [41]. Indeed, medical therapy for stricture management is limited due to fibrotic nature. Endoscopic dilatation may prevent or delay the need for surgical resection or strictureplasty. Moreover, endoscopic balloon dilation should be performed to access the mucosa proximal to strictures and evaluate disease activity, that otherwise may be missed if we only relied on symptoms or biochemical markers [42]. Thus, it can provide adequate endoscopic therapy and adjust or optimize medical therapy.

Endoscopic balloon dilation may be used in Crohn's strictures of the gastric outlet, duodenum, colon, ileocolonic anastomosis and of the small bowel, if accessible [43]. It is performed using a through-the-scope balloon catheter, which is a simple and safe procedure (**Figure 4**). The dilation procedure is performed with monitoring of the pressure of the inflated balloon using a dilator with or without X-ray guidance. When performing endoscopic balloon dilation, forcible dilation to achieve a larger dilation diameter or pressure is not recommended, as it could lead to intestinal perforation. The length of the balloons for inflation is about 5 cm; therefore, stenoses longer than 5 cm are considered unsuitable for endoscopic balloon dilation. Moreover, intestinal strictures with deep ulcers and fistulous complications are contraindications for endoscopic dilatation. In case of long or inflammatory strictures, balloon dilation may significantly increase the risk of perforation [44]. Hence, inflammatory and ulcerative strictures should be primarily treated with medical therapy.

Over the last years, there is increasing evidence for endoscopic balloon dilation as a safe and minimally invasive effective method for the treatment of stricturing disease. In a retrospective single tertiary center study, Lopes et al. evaluated the long-term efficacy and safety of endoscopic balloon dilation in ileocolonic

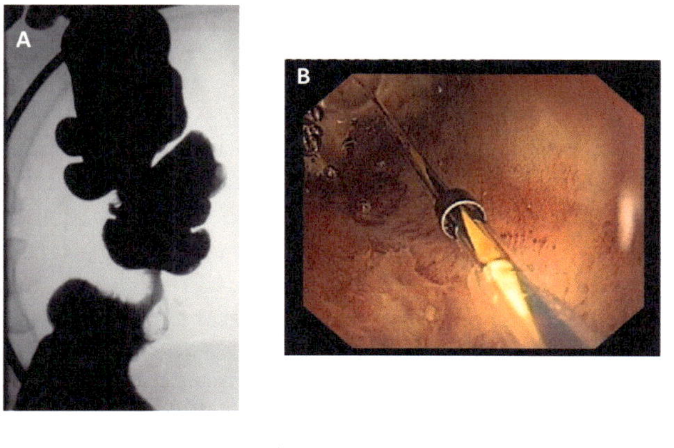

Figure 4.
A segment of short stenosis is delineated using injection of contrast via a catheter (A). A guide wire is inserted through the stenosis and a balloon is then advanced over the wire and carefully inflated (B).

strictures. The authors reported a technical success rate of 97.7% to anastomotic strictures and similar to non-anastomotic strictures (100%) without major adverse events (major bleeding and perforation) [40]. Endoscopic dilatation using balloon-assisted enteroscopy for small bowel strictures is almost the same as for ileocolonic strictures in terms of procedure and technique. However, there are some technical difficulties. In fact, it is not easy to stabilize the tip of the scope and to maintain a good visual field because of the limited space available, severe angulation, motility and adhesion in the small intestine. Nevertheless, the reported technical success rate is over 85% with a perforation rate of 1% [45, 46].

A key concern of endoscopic dilatation is the long-term outcome. Indeed, a recent study showed that 63% of patients with anastomotic strictures and 41% of those with non-anastomotic strictures required additional dilation over a 4.4-year period [40]. However, Sunada et al. reported that the surgery-free rate in 321 patients with CD who underwent endoscopic dilatation for small intestinal strictures was 87% and 78% at 1 and 3 years, respectively [47]. Similarly, a systematic review assessed the role of device-assisted enteroscopy in 581 small bowel dilatations, showing an 80% long-term success rate without the need for surgery during follow-up (2.5 years per patient) [48].

In conclusion, endoscopic balloon dilation is a feasible, simple, effective and safe procedure and an appropriate option for either delaying or preventing surgery, with the possibility of being repeated as needed.

To have a persistent effect over time and avoid the high risk of recurrence, a self-expanding metallic stent has been proposed [49]. Stenting appeared to be an effective technique in treating symptomatic CD intestinal strictures, however the procedure was associated with a high rate of spontaneous migrations and complications. More recently, an anti-migration, removable and shaped self-expandable metal stent is available. Attar et al. performed a real-life study to describe short- and long-term results of the removable anti-migration stent [50]. The authors showed that it was safe and effective in about half of patients and had an extremely low migration rate, with no perforation reported. In addition, the high success rate was close to that obtained with endoscopic balloon dilation, but without complications. Taking this into account, the placement of a transient metallic stent is a new minimally invasive alternative to the management of refractory anastomotic stricture of less than 5 cm, before considering a new surgery. The use of biodegradable instead of metal stents was recently evaluated in intestinal and colonic CD strictures. Although it was technically feasible, premature stent failure occurred in all of the patients, as well as side effects such as mucosal overgrowth and stent collapse [51].

3.2 Removal of impacted capsules

One problem of video capsule endoscopy in patients with suspected or known CD is the risk of impaction due to previously undiagnosed stenoses. One effort to overcome this difficulty was the development of the patency capsule. However, the successful passage of the patency capsule does not absolutely guarantee that intestinal obstruction will not occur during the passage of the video capsule. Similarly, some stenoses may not be detected by prior radiographic methods. Therefore, capsule impaction can occur.

A retained capsule, in general, does not cause obstruction. In fact, the capsule can remain in the small bowel for several months without causing symptoms. Thus, unless malignancy is strongly suspected, conservative or pharmaceutical intervention, namely with corticosteroids, are justified therapeutic options in the majority of cases [52].

When patients develop obstructive symptoms, they may have to undergo device-assisted enteroscopy or surgery. Push-and-pull enteroscopy using the double-balloon technique has proven to be extremely effective (90–100% of cases) and is considered the method of choice [53]. Surgery is an alternative procedure for removing impacted capsules, especially in those cases in which investigations unequivocally suggest the presence of neoplastic disease. The surgical intervention allows the removal of both the capsule and the pathology that caused capsule retention. In addition, intra-operative enteroscopy can be a useful tool to establish intra-luminal pathology like ulceration as a cause of retained endoscopic capsule.

Besides some cases of acute intestinal obstruction, there are only a few more complications reported in the literature due to a retained capsule. In fact, bowel perforation and capsule disintegration have already been reported, but only in case reports [54, 55].

3.3 Treatment of bleeding lesions

CD may be associated with mild gastrointestinal bleeding while major hemorrhage is a rare complication. In addition, a definitive bleeding site is not identified in most patients. In fact, hemorrhage is frequently attributed to diffuse areas of active inflammation [56]. The majority of bleeds originate from the ileum and colon and only a small number of episodes have been attributed to a jejunal or upper gastrointestinal source.

Initial management of major hemorrhage should always include primary resuscitation, as in any individual with a significant gastrointestinal bleed [57]. Once a patient is stabilized, diagnostic maneuvers are of primary importance. The site of bleeding can be identified by endoscopy, angiography or labeled red blood cell scans. However, clinicians should be aware that identifying a precise source of bleeding is difficult and salvage surgery may be necessary.

In the context of CD, urgent device-assisted enteroscopy for large-volume bleeding should be performed via the retrograde route, given the propensity of these conditions to involve the distal small bowel [52]. When it is identified, the source of bleeding is more commonly described as a deep ulcer eroding into a blood vessel and therapy may be attempted [56]. Endoscopy therapy includes thermocoagulation alone or a combination of epinephrine injection and bipolar coagulation [58]. Application of hemoclips may be compromised in the presence of inflamed and friable mucosa. On rare occasions, a large pseudopolyp in the ileum or colon has been identified as the source of bleeding; polypectomy should be performed in these cases. Although endoscopic therapy can stop acute bleeding, it does not promote mucosal healing and therefore cannot prevent rebleeding. In fact, the risk of rebleeding associated with endoscopic hemostasis is about 50% [56]. Thus, therapies that can induce and maintain mucosal healing are necessary to prevent rebleeding, such as anti-TNF agents.

Intraoperative enteroscopy may be the most reliable method to achieve a complete small bowel evaluation. It involves evaluation of the small bowel at laparotomy and may be performed orally, rectally or via an enterotomy. Upper endoscopes, colonoscopes, push enteroscopes and balloon-assisted scopes have all been used. Although it is highly invasive and associated with major complications, it may help in the identification of the bleeding source and in planning the optimal therapeutic intervention [59].

When CD is complicated by obscure bleeding, video capsule endoscopy and device-assisted endoscopy may identify and treat the bleeding source beyond the reach of standard endoscopes [1]. In fact, video capsule endoscopy has a fundamental role in diagnosing obscure gastrointestinal bleeding in patients with CD. It has been found to be superior to push enteroscopy and small bowel radiography. Video capsule endoscopy should be performed immediately after a negative upper and lower endoscopy as a screening method. The results of video capsule endoscopy should guide the use of device-assisted endoscopy, which aims at both the confirmation and treatment of the detected lesions.

3.4 Intralesional injection

Although local injection of immunomodulatory drugs like corticosteroids and infliximab CD stricture may look like an attractive therapeutic strategy [60], the available evidence is inconsistent. Some studies have shown benefit of intralesional injection of triamcinolone [61] and infliximab [62] at the time of balloon dilatation of CD. On the other hand, East et al. compared local quadrantic injection of triamcinolone after endoscopic balloon dilatation of Crohn's ileocolonic anastomotic strictures vs. saline placebo and showed that a single treatment of intrastricture triamcinolone injection did not reduce the time to redilatation [63]. Moreover, there was a trend toward a worse outcome. Similarly, Atreja et al. reported that intralesional steroid or biologics injection did not decrease the need for re-intervention or surgery for either primary or anastomotic strictures [64]. Until now, there is no strong evidence supporting the injection of drugs at the site of strictures and larger series are needed to evaluate the real effectiveness of these techniques in the treatment of patients with obstructive strictures.

4. Postoperative recurrence

In the natural history of CD, intestinal resection is unavoidable in a significant proportion of patients. The majority of individuals will develop disease recurrence at or above the anastomosis, which usually occurs within a few weeks to months after ileocolonic resection [65].

Diagnosis of postoperative recurrence is based on clinical symptoms, serum and fecal markers, radiological and endoscopic findings. Nevertheless, ileocolonoscopy remains the gold standard, by defining the presence and severity of morphological recurrence [41]. It is recommended within the first 6 to 12 months after surgery, when treatment decisions may be affected. In fact, endoscopic recurrence usually precedes clinical recurrence and severe endoscopic recurrence predicts a poor prognosis. Rutgeerts et al. developed an endoscopic scoring system to assess postoperative recurrence in patients having ileocolonic resection [66]. The patients were stratified into five groups according to the endoscopic severity (**Table 5**). An

Rutgeerts´ score	Endoscopic description of findings
i0	No lesions
i1	≤5 aphthous ulcers
i2	>5 aphthous ulcers with normal intervening mucosa, skip areas of larger lesions or lesions confined to ileocolonic anastomosis
i3	Diffuse aphthous ileitis with diffusely inflamed mucosa
i4	Diffuse inflammation with large ulcers, nodules and/or narrowing

Table 5.
Rutgeerts´ score. Postoperative recurrence: Rutgeerts score = i2-i4.

endoscopic score of i0 or i1 correlated with a low risk of endoscopic progression and had clinical recurrence rates of less than 10% over 10 years. An endoscopic score of i2 or above suggests mucosal inflammation and should prompt considered treatment escalation [14]. However, it is important to note that the i2 category, including aphthous lesions in the terminal ileum as well as ileocolonic anastomosis lesions, had a heterogeneous recurrence risk. Therefore, a modified Rutgeerts' score has recently emerged in which i2 is subdivided into i2a for lesions confined to the ileocolonic anastomosis, including anastomotic stenosis, and i2b for more than 5 aphthous ulcers or larger lesions, with normal mucosa in between, in the neoterminal ileum, with or without anastomotic lesions [67]. With this modified score, stenosis and/or ulceration of the anastomosis, which might simply be related to ischemia or staples, do not define recurrent disease and have no prognostic or therapeutic implications [68]. Thus, possible confounding factors for recurrent disease are overcome with this score.

Video capsule endoscopy can also be used to assess postoperative recurrence of CD and should be considered if ileocolonoscopy is contraindicated or unsuccessful. Video capsule endoscopy may identify lesions in the small bowel that have not been detected by ileocolonoscopy after ileocolic resection. An important advantage of capsule endoscopy is the ability to detect proximal small bowel recurrence. However, patency capsule evaluation is recommended before capsule endoscopy to minimize the risk of retention.

5. Small bowel malignancy

Patients with CD are at an increased risk of developing malignancy, which is more frequent in the CD-affected colon. However, those with small bowel involvement may also develop cancer, which can be difficult to diagnose. In fact, compared with an age-matched population, patients with CD have an 18-fold increased incidence of small bowel malignancy and only a minority are detected at an early stage [69]. Adenocarcinoma is the most common form of all small bowel cancer. Prognosis of small bowel adenocarcinoma is poor and the mortality at 1 and 2 years ranges from 30–60% dependent on the stage of cancer [70].

Early detection of small bowel carcinoma remains a problem. Radiological imaging and video capsule endoscopy could potentially detect malignancies at an early stage. However, differentiation between inflammatory stenosis and cancer is difficult. In these cases, device-assisted enteroscopy should be performed to direct visualization and tissue sampling. Furthermore, these procedures are not routinely used for screening asymptomatic individuals. Therefore, every patient who has a change of symptoms should perform further exams as this might be an indicator of malignancy [69]. Moreover, most of the small bowel carcinoma in CD is located in strictures, so the endoscopist should have a low threshold for taking biopsies before endoscopic balloon dilatation [71].

6. Conclusions

Endoscopy has major implications for diagnosis, classification, therapeutic decision and prognosis of CD. Ileocolonoscopy with biopsy is the first-line exam for suspected CD. However, the small bowel is one of the most affected areas by inflammation, which may skip the terminal ileum and not be detected by ileoscopy. In fact, small intestine involvement is more difficult to assess by conventional endoscopy. In addition, radiological examinations, including both magnetic resonance imaging and computed tomography, may not detect disease of the small bowel, especially in mild lesions.

Until a decade ago, mucosal visualization of the small intestine was limited to the reach of the push enteroscope. The advent of video capsule endoscopy and device-assisted endoscopy is revolutionizing small bowel CD diagnosis and treatment. In fact, these techniques allowed direct visualization of the entire small intestine, which would alter patient management, especially in those with inconclusive results from conventional studies. Device-assisted endoscopy has also the ability to obtain biopsies for histopathology and the potential for therapeutic intervention. Finally, video capsule endoscopy and device-assisted endoscopy play an important role in assessing response to therapy.

Conflict of interest

The authors declare no conflict of interest.

Author details

Isabel Garrido[1,2]*, Susana Lopes[1,2] and Guilherme Macedo[1,2]

1 Gastroenterology and Hepatology Department, Centro Hospitalar Universitário de São João, Porto, Portugal

2 World Gastroenterology Organization (WGO) Porto Training Center, Porto, Portugal

*Address all correspondence to: isabelmng@hotmail.com

IntechOpen

© 2021 The Author(s). Licensee IntechOpen. This chapter is distributed under the terms of the Creative Commons Attribution License (http://creativecommons.org/licenses/by/3.0), which permits unrestricted use, distribution, and reproduction in any medium, provided the original work is properly cited.

References

[1] Rubin DT, Ananthakrishnan AN, Siegel CA, Sauer BG, Long MD. ACG Clinical Guideline: Ulcerative Colitis in Adults. Am J Gastroenterol. 2019;114(3):384-413.

[2] Lashner B. Clinical features, laboratory findings, and course of Crohn's disease. In: Kirsner JV (ed) Inflammatory bowel disease. 5th ed. Philadelphia: Saunders. 2000: 305-314.

[3] Hall B, Holleran G, McNamara D. Small bowel Crohn's disease: an emerging disease phenotype? Dig Dis. 2015;33:42-51.

[4] Bourreille A, Ignjatovic A, Aabakken L, Loftus EV Jr, Eliakim R, Pennazio M, et al. World Organisation of Digestive Endoscopy (OMED) and the European Crohn's and Colitis Organisation (ECCO). Role of small-bowel endoscopy in the management of patients with inflammatory bowel disease: an international OMED-ECCO consensus. Endoscopy. 2009;41(7):618-637.

[5] Gomollón F, Dignass A, Annese V, Tilg H, Van Assche G, Lindsay JO, et al. ECCO. 3rd European Evidence-based Consensus on the Diagnosis and Management of Crohn's Disease 2016: Part 1: Diagnosis and Medical Management. J Crohns Colitis. 2017;11(1):3-25.

[6] Cherian S, Singh P. Is routine ileoscopy useful? An observational study of procedure times, diagnostic yield, and learning curve. Am J Gastroenterol. 2004;99:2324-2329.

[7] Lichtenstein GR, Loftus EV, Isaacs KL, Regueiro MD, Gerson LB, Sands BE. ACG Clinical Guideline: Management of Crohn's Disease in Adults. Am J Gastroenterol. 2018 Apr;113(4):481-517.

[8] Mary JY, Modigliani R. Development and validation of an endoscopic index of the severity for Crohn's disease: a prospective multicentre study. Groupe d'Etudes Therapeutiques des Affections Inflammatoires du Tube Digestif (GETAID). Gut. 1989;30:983-989.

[9] Daperno M, D'Haens G, Van Assche G, Baert F, Bulois P, Maunoury V, et al. Development and validation of a new, simplified endoscopic activity score for Crohn's disease: the SES-Crohn's Disease. Gastrointest Endosc. 2004;60:505-512.

[10] Samuel S, Bruining DH, Loftus EV Jr, Becker B, Fletcher JG, Mandrekar JN , et al. Endoscopic skipping of the distal terminal ileum in Crohn's disease can lead to negative results from ileocolonoscopy. Clin Gastroenterol Hepatol. 2012;10:1253-1259.

[11] Schwartzberg DM, Brandstetter S, Grucela AL. Crohn's disease of the esophagus, duodenum, and stomach. Clin Colon Rectal Surg. 2019;32:231-242.

[12] Annunziata M, Caviglia R, Papparella LG, Cicala M. Upper gastrointestinal involvement of Crohn's disease: a prospective study on the role of upper endoscopy in the diagnostic work-up. Dig Dis Sci. 2012;57:1618-1623.

[13] Witte AM, Veenendaal RA, Van Hogezand RA, Verspaget HW, Lamers CB. Crohn's disease of the upper gastrointestinal tract: the value of endoscopic examination. Scand J Gastroenterol Suppl. 1998;225:100-105.

[14] Lamb CA, Kennedy NA, Raine T, Hendy PA, Smith PJ, Limdi JK, et al. British Society of Gastroenterology consensus guidelines on the management of inflammatory bowel disease in adults. Gut. 2019;68(Suppl 3): s1-s106.

[15] Robertson KD, Singh R. Capsule Endoscopy [Internet]. 2020. Available from: https://www.ncbi.nlm.nih.gov/books/NBK482306/.

[16] ASGE Technology Committee, Wang A, Banerjee S, Barth BA, Bhat YM, Chauhan S, et al. Wireless capsule endoscopy. Gastrointest Endosc. 2013 Dec;78(6):805-815.

[17] Spada C, Hassan C, Galmiche JP, Neuhaus H, Dumonceau JM, Adler S, et al. European Society of Gastrointestinal Endoscopy. Colon capsule endoscopy: European Society of Gastrointestinal Endoscopy (ESGE) Guideline. Endoscopy. 2012 May;44(5):527-536.

[18] Rodrigues-Pinto E, Cardoso H, Rosa B, Santos-Antunes J, Rodrigues S, Marques M, et al. Development of a predictive model of Crohn's disease proximal small bowel involvement in capsule endoscopy evaluation. Endosc Int Open. 2016;4(6):E631–E636.

[19] Dionisio P, Gurudu S, Leighton JA, Leontiadis GI, Fleischer DE, Hara AK, et al. Capsule endoscopy has a significantly higher diagnostic yield in patients with suspected and established small-bowel Crohn's disease: a meta-analysis. Am J Gastroenterol. 2010;105:1240-1248.

[20] Hall B, Holleran G, Costigan D, McNamara D. Capsule endoscopy: high negative predictive value in the long term despite a low diagnostic yield in patients with suspected Crohn's disease. United European Gastroenterology J. 2013;1:461-468.

[21] Solem CA, Loftus EV Jr, Fletcher JG, Baron TH, Gostout CJ, Petersen BT, et al. Small-bowel imaging in Crohn's disease: a prospective, blinded, 4-way comparison trial. Gastrointest Endosc. 2008;68:255-266.

[22] Mow WS, Lo SK,Targan SR, Dubinsky MC, Treyzon L, Abreu-Martin MT, et al. Initial experience with wireless capsule enteroscopy in the diagnosis and management of inflammatory bowel disease. Clin Gastroenterol Hepatol. 2004;2:31-40.

[23] Niv Y, Ilani S, Levi Z, Hershkowitz M, Niv E, Fireman Z, et al. Validation of the Capsule Endoscopy Crohn's Disease Activity Index [CECDAI or Niv score]: a multicenter prospective study. Endoscopy. 2012;44:21-26.

[24] Monteiro S, Boal Carvalho P, Dias de Castro F, Magalhães J, Machado F, Moreira MJ, et al. Capsule endoscopy: diagnostic accuracy of Lewis score in patients with suspected Crohn's disease. Inflamm Bowel Dis. 2015;21:2241-2246.

[25] Kopylov U, Nemeth A, Koulaouzidis A, Makins R, Wild G, Afif W, et al. Small bowel capsule endoscopy in the management of established Crohn's disease: clinical impact, safety, and correlation with inflammatory biomarkers. Inflamm Bowel Dis. 2015;21:93-100.

[26] Santos-AntunesJ, CardosoH, LopesS, Marques M, Nunes AC, Macedo G. Capsule enteroscopy is useful for the therapeutic management of Crohn's disease. World J Gastroenterol. 2015;21(44):12660-12666.

[27] Park S, Ye B, Kim KO, Park CH, Lee WS, Jang BI, et al. Guidelines for video capsule endoscopy: emphasis on Crohn's disease . Clin Endosc. 2015;48:128-135.

[28] Nemeth A, Kopylov U, Koulaouzidis A, Wurm Johansson G, Thorlacius H, Amre D, et al. Use of patency capsule in patients with established Crohn's disease. Endoscopy. 2016;48:373-379.

[29] Dubcenco E, Jeejeebhoy KN, Petroniene R, Tang SJ, Zalev AH, Gardiner GW, et al. Capsule endoscopy findings in patients with established and

suspected small-bowel Crohn's disease: correlation with radiologic, endoscopic, and histologic findings. Gastrointest Endosc. 2005;62:538-544.

[30] Repici A, Barbon V, De Angelis C, Luigiano C, De Caro G, Hervoso C, et al. Acute small-bowel perforation secondary to capsule endoscopy. Gastrointest Endosc. 2008;67:180-183.

[31] Schneider M, Höllerich J, Beyna T. Device-assisted enteroscopy: A review of available techniques and upcoming new technologies. World J Gastroenterol. 2019;25(27):3538-3545.

[32] Yamamoto H, Sekine Y, Sato Y, Higashizawa T, Miyata T, Iino S, et al. Total enteroscopy with a nonsurgical steerable double-balloon method. Gastrointest Endosc. 2001;53:216-220.

[33] Neuhaus H, Beyna T, Schneider M, Devière J. Novel motorized spiral enteroscopy: first clinical case. VideoGIE 2016;1:32-33.

[34] Beyna T, Arvanitakis M, Schneider M, Gerges C, Böing D, Devière J, et al. Motorised spiral enteroscopy: first prospective clinical feasibility study. Gut. 2021 Feb;70(2):261-267.

[35] Seiderer J, Herrmann K, Diepolder H, Schoenberg SO, Wagner AC, Göke B, et al. Double-balloon enteroscopy versus magnetic resonance enteroclysis in diagnosing suspected small-bowel Crohn's disease: results of a pilot study. Scand J Gastroenterol. 2007;42:1376-1385.

[36] Tontini G, Vecchi M, Neurath M, Neumann H. Advanced endoscopic imaging techniques in Crohn's disease. J Crohns Colitis. 2014;8:261-269.

[37] Mensink PB, Aktas H, Zelinkova Z, West RL, Kuipers EJ, van der Woude CJ. Impact of double-balloon enteroscopy findings on the management of Crohn's disease. Scand J Gastroenterol. 2010;45:483-489.

[38] Gerson L, Chiorean M, Tokar J, Decker A, Cave D, BouHaidar D, et al. Complications associated with double balloon enteroscopy: the US experience. Am J Gastroenterol. 2008; 103:S109–S110.

[39] Navaneethan U, Vargo JJ, Menon KV, Sanaka MR, Tsai CJ. Impact of balloon-assisted enteroscopy on the diagnosis and management of suspected and established small bowel Crohn's disease. Endosc Int Open. 2014;2:E201–E206.

[40] Lopes S, Rodrigues-Pinto E, Andrade P, Afonso J, Baron TH, Magro F, et al. Endoscopic balloon dilation of Crohn's disease strictures-safety, efficacy and clinical impact. World J Gastroenterol. 2017;23(41):7397-7406.

[41] Gionchetti P, Dignass A, Danese S, Magro Dias FJ, Rogler G, Lakatos PL, et al. ECCO. 3rd European Evidence-based Consensus on the Diagnosis and Management of Crohn's Disease 2016: Part 2: Surgical Management and Special Situations. J Crohns Colitis. 2017;11(2):135-149.

[42] Lopes S, Andrade P, Rodrigues-Pinto E, Afonso J, Macedo G, Magro F. Fecal marker levels as predictors of need for endoscopic balloon dilation in Crohn's disease patients with anastomotic strictures. World J Gastroenterol. 2017;23(35):6482-6490.

[43] Hirai F. Current status of endoscopic balloon dilation for Crohn's disease. Intest Res. 2017;15(2):166-173.

[44] Sunada K, Yamamoto H, Yano T, Sugano K. Advances in the diagnosis and treatment of small bowel lesions in Crohn's disease using double-balloon endoscopy. Ther Adv Gastroenterol. 2009;2:357-366.

[45] Rahman A, Ross A, Leighton JA, Schembre D, Gerson L, Lo SK, et al. Double-balloon enteroscopy in Crohn's disease: findings and impact on management in a multicenter retrospective study. Gastrointest Endosc. 2015;82(1):102-107.

[46] Halloran BP, Jamil LH, Lo SK, Reeson M, Vasiliauskas EA, Targan S, et al. Double-Balloon Endoscopy in Crohn Disease: A Tertiary Referral Center Experience. Inflamm Bowel Dis. 2020:izaa287.

[47] Sunada K, Shinozaki S, Nagayama M, Yano T, Takezawa T, Ino Y, et al. Long-term Outcomes in Patients with Small Intestinal Strictures Secondary to Crohn's Disease After Double-balloon Endoscopy-assisted Balloon Dilation. Inflamm Bowel Dis. 2016;22(2):380-386.

[48] Baars JE, Theyventhiran R, Aepli P, Saxena P, Kaffes AJ. Double-balloon enteroscopy-assisted dilatation avoids surgery for small bowel strictures: a systematic review. World J Gastroenterol. 2017;23(December (45)):8073-81.

[49] Attar A, Maunoury V, Vahedi K, Vernier-Massouille G, Vida S, Bulois P, et al. Safety and efficacy of extractible self-expandable metal stents in the treatment of Crohn's disease intestinal strictures: A prospective pilot study. Inflamm Bowel Dis. 2012;18(10):1849-1854.

[50] Attar A, Branche J, Coron E, Privat J, Caillo L, Chevaux JB, et al. An Anti-Migration Self-Expandable and Removable Metal Stent for Crohn's Disease Strictures: A Nationwide Study From the Getaid and the Sfed. J Crohns Colitis. 2020:jjaa208.

[51] Karstensen JG, Christensen KR, Brynskov J, Rønholt C, Vilmann P, Hendel J. Biodegradable stents for the treatment of bowel strictures in Crohn's disease: technical results and challenges. Endosc Int Open. 2016.;4(3):E296–E300.

[52] Rondonotti E, Spada C, Adler S, May A, Despott EJ, Koulaouzidis A, et al. Small-bowel capsule endoscopy and device-assisted enteroscopy for diagnosis and treatment of small-bowel disorders: European Society of Gastrointestinal Endoscopy (ESGE) Technical Review. Endoscopy. 2018;50(4):423-446.

[53] Mitsui K, Fujimori S, Tanaka S, Ehara A, Omori J, Akimoto N, et al. Retrieval of retained capsule endoscopy at small bowel stricture by double-balloon endoscopy significantly decreases surgical treatment. J Clin Gastroenterol. 2016;50:141-146.

[54] Gonzalez Carro P, Picazo Yuste J, Fernández Díez S, Pérez Roldán F, Roncero García-Escribano O. Intestinal perforation due to retained wireless capsule endoscope. Endoscopy. 2005;37:684.

[55] Fry LC, De Petris G, Swain JM, Fleischer DE. Impaction and fracture of a video capsule in the small bowel requiring laparotomy for removal of the capsule fragments. Endoscopy. 2005;37:674-676.

[56] Podugu A, Tandon K, Castro FJ. Crohn's disease presenting as acute gastrointestinal hemorrhage. World J Gastroenterol. 2016;22(16):4073-4078.

[57] Korzenik JR. Massive Lower Gastrointestinal Hemorrhage in Crohn's Disease. Curr Treat Options Gastroenterol. 2000 Jun;3(3):211-216.

[58] Belaiche J, Louis E, D'Haens G, Cabooter M, Naegels S, De Vos M, et al. Acute lower gastrointestinal bleeding in Crohn's disease: characteristics of a unique series of 34 patients. Belgian IBD Research Group. Am J Gastroenterol. 1999;94:2177-2181.

[59] Daperno M, Sostegni R, Rocca R. Lower gastrointestinal bleeding in Crohn's disease: how (un-)common is it and how to tackle it? Dig Liver Dis. 2012;44:721-722.

[60] Kochhar R, Poornachandra KS. Intralesional steroid injection therapy in the management of resistant gastrointestinal strictures. World J Gastrointest Endosc. 2010;2:61-68.

[61] Brooker JC, Beckett CG, Saunders BP, Benson MJ. Long-acting steroid injection after endoscopic dilation of anastomotic Crohn's strictures may improve the outcome: a retrospective case series. Endoscopy. 2003;35:333-337.

[62] Hendel J, Karstensen JG, Vilmann P. Serial intralesional injections of infliximab in small bowel Crohn's strictures are feasible and might lower inflammation. United European Gastroenterol J. 2014;2(5):406-412.

[63] East JE, Brooker JC, Rutter MD, Saunders BP. A pilot study of intrastricture steroid versus placebo injection after balloon dilatation of Crohn's strictures. Clin Gastroenterol Hepatol. 2007;5:1065-1069.

[64] Atreja A, Aggarwal A, Dwivedi S, Rieder F, Lopez R, Lashner BA, et al. Safety and efficacy of endoscopic dilation for primary and anastomotic Crohn's disease strictures. J Crohns Colitis. 2014;8:392-400.

[65] Olaison G, Smedh K, Sjodahl R. Natural course of Crohn's disease after ileocolic resection: endoscopically visualised ileal ulcers preceding symptoms. Gut. 1992;33:331-335.

[66] Rutgeerts P, Geboes K, Vantrappen G, Beyls J, Kerremans R, Hiele M. Predictability of the postoperative course of Crohn's disease. Gastroenterology. 1990;99:956-963.

[67] Gecse K, Lowenberg M, Bossuyt P, Rutgeerts P, Vermeire S, Stitt S, et al. Sa1198 Agreement among experts in the endoscopic evaluation of postoperative recurrence in Crohn's disease using the Rutgeerts Score. Gastroenterology. 2014;146:S-227.

[68] Lopes S, Andrade P, Afonso J, Rodrigues-Pinto E, Dias CC, Macedo G, et al. Correlation Between Calprotectin and Modified Rutgeerts Score. Inflamm Bowel Dis. 2016;22(9):2173-2181.

[69] Laukoetter MG, Mennigen R, Hannig CM, Osada N, Rijcken E, Vowinkel T, et al. Intestinal cancer risk in Crohn's disease: a meta-analysis. J Gastrointest Surg. 2011;15(4):576-583.

[70] Rieder F, Latella G, Magro F, Yuksel ES, Higgins PD, Di Sabatino A, et al. European Crohn's and Colitis Organisation topical review on prediction, diagnosis and management of fibrostenosing Crohn's disease. J Crohns Colitis. 2016;10:873-885.

[71] Maaser C, Sturm A, Vavricka SR, Kucharzik T, Fiorino G, Annese V, et al. European Crohn's and Colitis Organisation [ECCO] and the European Society of Gastrointestinal and Abdominal Radiology [ESGAR]. ECCO-ESGAR Guideline for Diagnostic Assessment in IBD Part 1: Initial diagnosis, monitoring of known IBD, detection of complications. J Crohns Colitis. 2019;13(2):144-164.

Chapter 4

Role of Small Bowel Endoscopy in Diagnosis and Management of Inflammatory Bowel Disease: Current Perspective

Partha Pal, D. Nageshwar Reddy and Zaheer Nabi

Abstract

The evaluation of small bowel in inflammatory bowel disease (IBD) is mainly performed in cases with newly diagnosed or suspected Crohn's disease (CD). The available modalities for small bowel evaluation include radiological imaging (barium meal follow through, magnetic resonance enteroclysis, computed tomography enteroclysis) and small bowel endoscopy also known as enteroscopy. The main advantage of small bowel endoscopy over radiological imaging is that it allows for obtaining biopsy specimen required for histological confirmation of the diagnosis. Various endoscopic modalities for endoscopic evaluation of small bowel include push enteroscopy and device assisted enteroscopy (DAE). Push enteroscopy allows only limited evaluation of proximal small bowel. Therefore, DAE is generally preferred over push enteroscopy for small bowel evaluation. DAE includes single balloon enteroscopy, double balloon enteroscopy, and spiral enteroscopy. The available literature suggests that there is no significant difference in the diagnostic yield among the available DAE devices. Therefore, the choice of DAE is largely dependent on the availability as well as local expertise. More recently, motorised spiral enteroscopy has been introduced. The main advantage of this novel DAE is ease of use with the possibility of evaluating the entire small bowel via per-oral route. However, the data regarding the use of motorised spiral enteroscopy is limited and comparative trials are required in future.

Keywords: small bowel, endoscopy, advances

1. Introduction

Evaluation of the small bowel in inflammatory bowel disease (IBD) is indicated primarily in patients with newly diagnosed or suspected Crohn's disease (CD) [1]. Small bowel evaluation can also be helpful in IBD- unclassified (IBD-U) who can be re-classified as CD in a significant number of cases. Small bowel evaluation in these settings can be done by imaging (barium meal follow through - BMFT, magnetic resonance enterography/enteroclysis - MRE, computed tomography enterography/ enteroclysis -CTE) or by endoscopy. Small bowel endoscopy refers to endoluminal examination of the small bowel. Endoscopic evaluation of small bowel can be done by small bowel video capsule endoscopy (VCE) (**Figure 1A**), push enteroscopy,

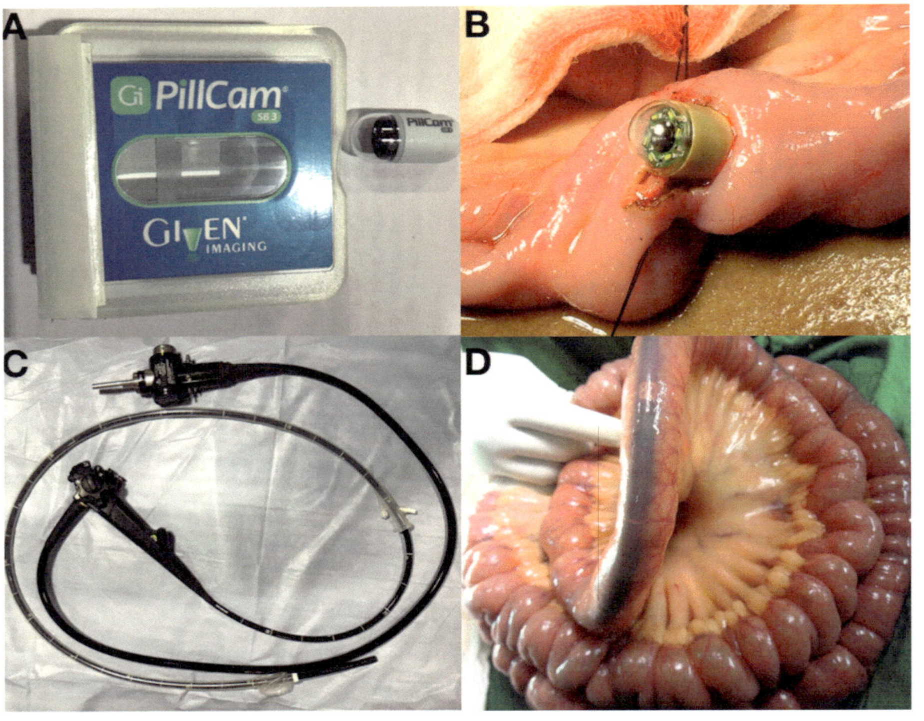

Figure 1.
Types of small bowel endoscopy. A. Video capsule endoscopy for small bowel (PillCam, given imaging ltd., Yokñeam Illit, Isareal), B. retained capsule removed at laparotomy, C. single balloon enteroscope (SIF-Q180, Olympus, Tokyo, Japan) with overture and balloon, D. intra-operative enteroscopy being performed at laparotomy.

device assisted enteroscopy (DAE) (which includes single balloon enteroscopy-SBE, double balloon enteroscopy - DBE, spiral enteroscopy, novel motorised spiral enteroscopy - NMSE and balloon guided endoscopy) (**Figure 1C**) and intra-operative enteroscopy (IOE) (**Figure 1D**) [2].

In about two-thirds of patients with CD, small bowel is involved at diagnosis [3]. Among them, 90% have involvement of terminal ileum. Skip lesions in terminal ileum can lead to false negative results. So for diagnosis of suspected CD, ileo-colonoscopy is the first line investigation [4]. VCE is the preferred initial diagnostic modality in cases with suspected CD and negative ileo-colonoscopy in the absence of obstructive symptoms or known stenosis. However, small bowel evaluation is warranted in all newly diagnosed cases of CD as small bowel is involved in every 2 out of 3 CD patients and the involvement can be discontinuous. In this scenario, cross sectional imaging (CTE/MRE) is preferred over VCE due to its potential to assess transmural and extra-luminal disease. VCE is indicated subsequently if cross sectional imaging is non-contributory. Patients with suspected small bowel involvement on cross sectional imaging or VCE, DAE with small bowel biopsy can provide definitive evidence of CD. Additionally, DAE is recommended for treatment of small bowel strictures amenable for endoscopic therapy, small bowel bleeding and retrieval of foreign bodies/retained capsule. For assessing the response to therapy in small bowel CD, VCE can be considered in primarily non-stricturing CD [2]. Hence, small bowel endoscopy has major implications in the diagnosis and classification, therapeutic decision making and altering treatment outcomes in IBD [5].

2. Indications of SB endoscopy in IBD

The Indications of small bowel endoscopy in IBD are [2, 5]

1. Suspicion of isolated small bowel CD,

2. Assessment of small bowel involvement in patients with confirmed CD,

3. Assessment for post-operative recurrence of CD in small bowel after ileo-colonic resection [6],

4. Small bowel assessment in IBD-U,

5. As a therapeutic tool in small bowel CD (stricture dilatation, retained capsule or foreign body retrieval, haemostasis for small bowel bleed).

6. Evaluation of anaemia and unexplained abdominal symptoms in cases with ulcerative colitis (UC) [7],

7. To rule out CD prior to elective colectomy in refractory UC,

8. Investigate anaemia after ileal pouch anal anastomosis (IPAA) in UC [8].

3. Role of small bowel endoscopy in suspected CD

There is no single reference standard for diagnosis of CD. Constellation of clinical history, biochemical and stool biomarkers, endoscopy, cross sectional imaging and histopathology is required for diagnosis of CD [9, 10]. Upto 30% CD patients have isolated small bowel disease. Improvement in endoscopic techniques (VCE, DAE, NMSE) as well as radiographic techniques (CTE/MRE) have revolutionised the diagnosis of small bowel CD [5]. However, options for histopathological confirmation in isolated CD is still limited, which is important in resource limited countries where infections (eg. tuberculosis) still predominate and needs to be excluded prior to initiation of therapy [11].

4. VCE in CD

The original VCE (PillCam, Given imaging Ltd., Yokñeam Illit, Isareal) (**Figure 1A**) was designed for visualisation of small bowel which has undergone many modifications such as higher image resolution and increasing diagnostic yield by faster adjustable frame rate and real time analysis capability [12].

4.1 VCE in suspected small bowel CD

European society of gastrointestinal endoscopy (ESGE) recommends VCE as the first line investigation in suspected small bowel CD in whom ileo-colonoscopy is negative in the absence of obstructive symptoms/known stenosis (**Figure 2**) [2]. This recommendation is based on the high sensitivity and negative predictive value (NPV)(ranging from 96–100%) of VCE in small bowel CD. However, the accuracy and diagnostic yield of VCE in suspected CD could not be determined precisely due

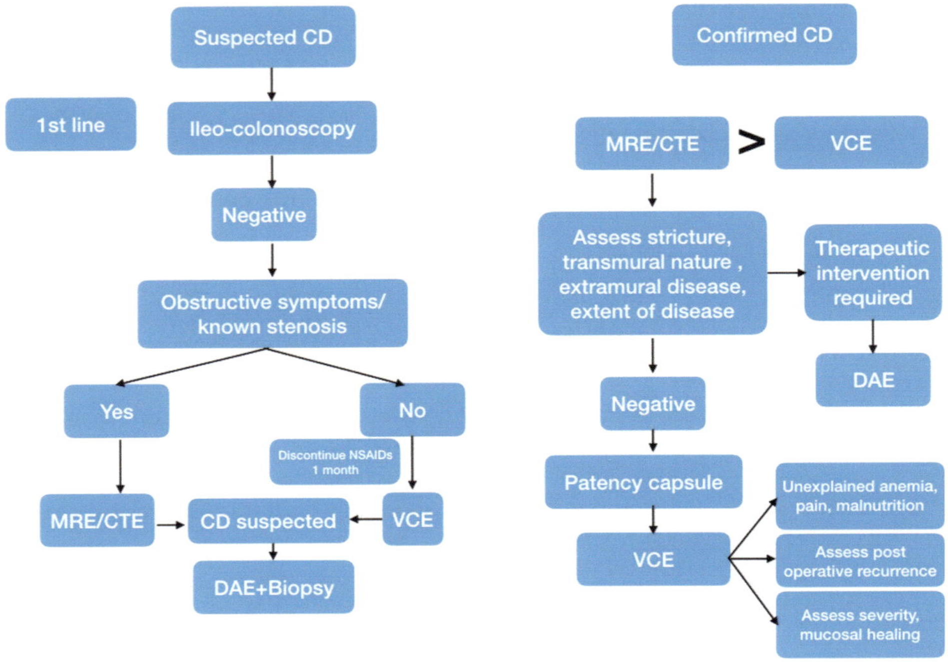

Figure 2.
Algorithm for small bowel evaluation in a suspected or known case of Crohn's disease (CD). DAE- device assisted enteroscopy, MRE- magnetic resonance enteroclysis, CTE- computed tomography enteroclysis, VCE- video capsule endoscopy.

to lack of gold standard for CD diagnosis and non-specific nature of findings on VCE. The lesions detected in VCE can be due to other causes such as non-steroidal anti-inflammatory drugs (NSAIDs) use, cryptogenic multifocal ulcerated stenosing enteritis, intestine tuberculosis, lymphoma, small bowel malignancy and intestinal Behcet's disease. VCE findings like small mucosal breaks or erosions are seen in upto 20% of normal individuals. Hence, the positive predictive value (PPV) of VCE is dependent on the patient population and criteria for CD diagnosis in VCE [13]. Lewis score (LS) can be helpful in this regard. LS <135 signifies clinically non-significant lesion. LS > 135 detects significant small bowel lesion with 83.2% overall accuracy. LS between 135–790 is mild and > 790 indicates moderate to severe disease [14].

4.2 VCE in confirmed small bowel CD

In patients with confirmed CD on ileo-colonoscopy, further small bowel evaluation is warranted irrespective of findings on ileo-colonoscopy (**Figure 2**). In this regard, dedicated small bowel cross sectional imaging (CTE/MRE) scores over VCE due to the ability to assess strictures, transmural involvement, intra-abdominal complications (abscess/fistula), extra-intestinal manifestations and anatomical distribution of the disease [2]. VCE is recommended subsequently if cross sectional imaging is non-contributory and if VCE findings could influence management. Small bowel CD only visible on VCE with normal cross sectional imaging is a new entity. A recent retrospective study have showed that it has a more favourable course compared to general CD with lower risk of complicated disease and requirement of step up therapy [15]. If VCE is indicated in confirmed CD, functional patency of the bowel should be confirmed with patency capsule given high rate of capsule retention in known CD (upto 13%) [2, 16]. In 27–40% cases, CTE/MRE finding suggestive of small bowel stricture may preclude VCE. However, not all strictures cause significant mechanical obstruction and patency capsule can be useful in this scenario [5]. The negative predictive value for ruling out a stricture is not different between patency capsule and non-enteroclysis small bowel radiologic examination according to a retrospective study [17].

Meta-analysis by Dionisio et al. have shown that VCE was superior to small bowel follow through (SBFT)/small bowel enteroclysis (36%) and CTE (39%) with higher diagnostic yield (71%). In comparison, the diagnostic yield of VCE was inferior to MRE (79%) [18]. However, VCE is superior to CTE/MRE in diagnosing proximal small bowel lesions and detects small bowel lesions in 50% patients with previously diagnosed ileal CD [19]. VCE can also be considered when symptoms suggestive of small bowel disease (anaemia, malnutrition, pain abdomen) do not correlate with imaging findings. In a retrospective study, VCE led to a change in management in 45% cases in these settings [19]. VCE can be helpful in suspected flares of CD, where small bowel cross sectional imaging is normal [20].

Another indication of VCE is longitudinal follow up of small bowel CD to see for response to therapy such as mucosal healing [2]. Endoscopic mucosal healing has emerged as an important therapeutic target in CD as it can predict future relapses. In a prospective, observational cohort study from Israeli IBD Research Nucleus (IIRN) it was shown that VCE predicted both short and long term flare risk in patients with quiescent, asymptomatic CD. Increment in Lewis score was better than MRE global score [21]. Similarly, in a prospective study including paediatric CD patients, VCE based treat to target strategy significantly increased number of patients achieving mucosal healing or deep remission [22].

Capsule retention in established CD can be treated with an observant, conservative trial of medical therapy using steroids and/or immunomodulators failing which endoscopic retrieval with DAE can be be attempted. Even in case of failure of endoscopic retrieval of retained capsule, most of the patients can be managed conservatively in the absence of obstructive symptoms [23]. Only a minority finally require surgery (**Figure 1B**). In a retrospective study of more than 2300 patients, among 301 CD patients (196 with confirmed small bowel involvement), 5 (1.6%) developed capsule retention but only 2 required surgical intervention [24].

4.3 Role of VCE scores to evaluate CD

Objective clinical activity scores are recommended to assess disease severity, small bowel involvement and response to medical therapy [2]. However, it should be borne in mind that these scores are for assessing type, location and severity of small bowel involvement but not for diagnosis of small bowel CD. For diagnosis of small bowel CD, Mow et al. proposed a cut off of more than 3 ulcers which is widely used for diagnosis of CD and has modest positive predictive value (PPV): 50–70% [25]. This however does not give any idea about location, severity and other inflammatory features such as edema and stenosis [2, 13]. There are two widely used validated scores to assess severity of small bowel CD on VCE: the Lewis score (LS) and the Capsule endoscopy Crohn's disease activity index (CECDAI) (**Tables 1** and **2**) [26, 27]. LS is based upon distribution and presence of ulcers (**Figure 3A, B**), villous edema and stenosis (**Figure 3C**). CECDAI evaluates severity of inflammation, extent of disease and stenosis. Among the two, CECDAI is simpler and was shown to be more reflective for active small bowel inflammation than LS in a comparative study [28]. There is strong correlation between LS and CECDAI but only moderate correlation with stool biomarkers such as faecal calprotectin [29]. A study showed that LS between 135–790 was equivalent to 4.9–6.9 score in CECDAI [28].

Parameters	Number	Longitudinal extent	Descriptors
First tertile			
Villous appearance	Normal - 0 Edematous - 1	Short segment - 8 Long segment - 12 Whole tertile - 20	Single - 1 Patchy –14 Diffuse –17
Ulcer	None-0 Single-3 Few-5 Multiple - 10	Short segment - 5 Longsegment-10 Whole tertile - 15	< 1/4–9 1/4–1/2–12 >1/2–18
Second tertile			
Villous appearance	Normal - 0	Short segment - 8	Single - 1
	Edematous - 1	Long segment - 12	Patchy –14
		Whole tertile - 20	Diffuse - 17
Ulcer	None-0	Short segment - 5	<1/4–9
	Single - 3	Long segment - 10	1/4–1/2–12
	Few-5	Whole tertile - 15	>1/2–18
	Multiple - 10		
Third tertile			
Villous appearance	Normal - 0 Edematous - 1	Short segment - 8 Long segment - 12 Whole tertile - 20	Single - 1 Patchy –14 Diffuse –17
Ulcer	None-0 Single-3 Few-5 Multiple - 10	Short segment - 5 Longsegment-10 Whole tertile - 15	< 1/4–9 1/4–1/2–12 >1/2–18
Stenosis (rated for the whole study)			
Stenosis	None-0	Ulcerated - 24	Traversed - 7
	Single –14	Non-ulcerated - 2	Not traversed - 10
	Multiple - 20		

Table 1.
The Lewis score for the assessment of small bowel lesions using small bowel capsule Endoscopy [26].

In a retrospective study on patients with established CD, VCE led to treatment escalation in 45% patients. The indications of small bowel VCE were unexplained anaemia, discrepancy between symptoms and imaging, evaluation of full extent of CD to document mucosal healing [30]. Nevertheless, the risk of capsule retention even with normal cross sectional imaging study should be kept in mind in established CD prior to VCE and hence patency capsules are strongly recommended [12].

4.4 Role of patency capsule

Patency capsule use is strongly recommended in stablished CD prior to small bowel VCE to assess functional patency of small bowel. Patency capsule can be used selectively (in patients with symptoms of intestinal obstruction/history of intestinal obstruction or surgery/ patients with stricture on cross sectional imaging) or non-selectively (in all CD patients). A retrospective multi-center study have shown that the risk capsule retention was not significantly different with non-selective use (2.1%) compared to elective use (1.5%). But retention rate is as high as 11% after positive patency test [31].

CECDAI Scoring System		
CECDAI	**Proximal**	**Distal**
A. Inflammation score		
0 = None		
1 = Mild to moderate edema/hyperemia/denudation		
2 = Severe edema/hyperemia/denudation		
3 = Bleeding, exudate, aphthae, erosion, small ulcer (≥ 0.5 cm)		
4 = Moderate ulcer (0.5–2 cm), pseudopolyp		
5 = Large ulcer (2 cm)		
B. Extent of disease score		
0 = None		
1 = Focal disease (single segment)		
2 = Patchy disease (multiple segments)		
3 = Diffuse disease		
C. Narrowing (stricture)		
0 = None		
1 = Single-passed		
2 = Multiple-passed		
Segmental score = **A × B + C**		
Total score = **(A1 × B1 + C1) + (A2 × B2 + C2)**		

Table 2.
The capsule endoscopy Crohn's disease activity index (CECDAI) for the assessment of small bowel lesions using small bowel capsule Endoscopy [27].

Two types of patency capsules have been described: the Given patency capsule (M2A) and the Agile patency capsule. Agile capsule has two timer plugs compared to one timer plug in Given patency capsule. Agile capsule starts dissolving after 30 hours compared to 40–100 hours with Given patency capsule. Given capsule is composed of lactose whereas Agile capsule is composed of dissolvable components surrounding a small radio frequency identification tag which can be detectable by X ray [32, 33]. Rare cases of symptomatic intestinal occlusion have been reported with patency capsules [33, 34]. Agile capsule further reduces the risk of symptomatic intestinal obstruction. Hence, risk of symptomatic obstruction is minimal and patency capsules can be used safely. Most of the cases of abdominal pain due to obstruction is relieved by conservative measures with only a small minority requiring endoscopic or surgical intervention [33, 35].

Given unclear benefit of non-selective use of patency capsules in CD and high risk of capsule retention in CD, the use of patency capsule should be based on clinical history, imaging finding, clinician's discretion and availability.

4.5 Assessment of postoperative CD recurrence

Intestinal resection is eventually required in upto three fourth of CD patients after 20 years of disease [36]. Postoperative recurrence after ileo-colonic resection can occur in upto 70% patients after 20 years post surgery. Ileal lesions can be scored by Rutgreet's score at the first ileocolonoscopy (ideally at 6 months postoperatively) which help to predict post operative recurrence: i0, no lesions: i1—less

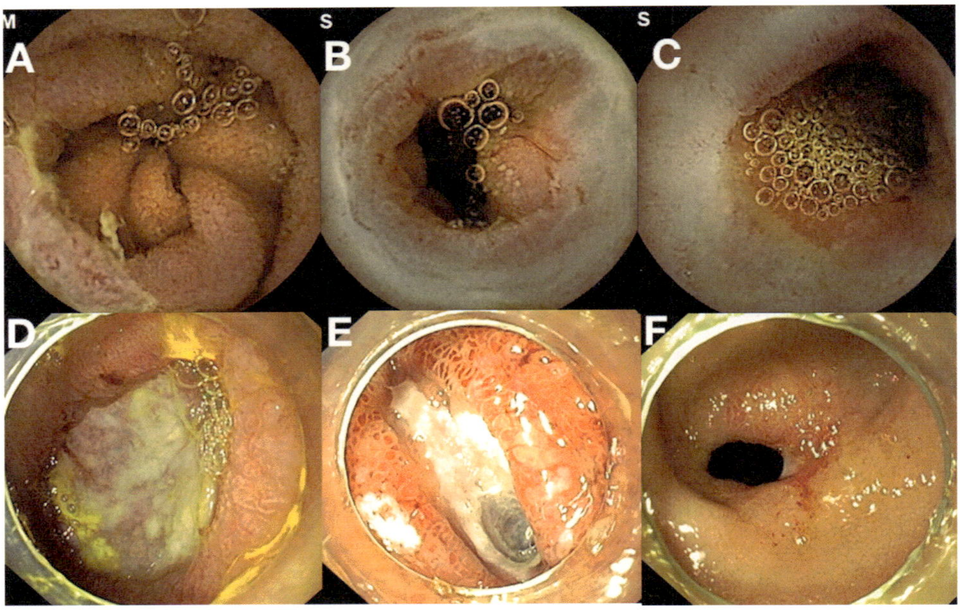

Figure 3.
Small bowel capsule endoscopy (A-C) and enteroscopy (D-F) in Crohn's disease (CD). A and B showing ulcers in CD, C. ulcerated stricture in CD, D. large deep ulcer in CD on device assisted enteroscopy (DAE), E. tight inflammatory stricture in CD, F. mildly inflamed stricture in CD on DAE.

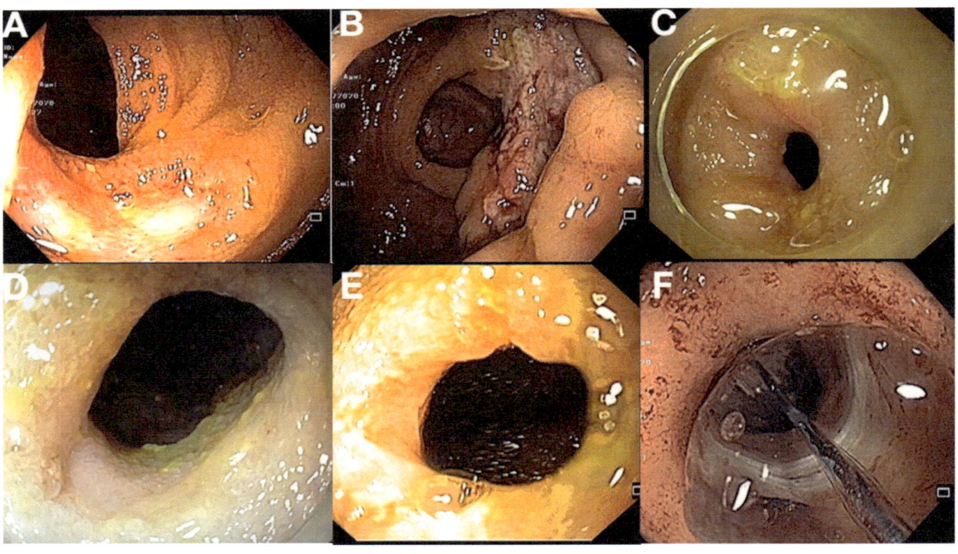

Figure 4.
Post-operative recurrence of Crohn's disease (CD) (A-B) and endoscopic management of CD strictures. A. Ileal recurrence of CD on ileoscopy. B. Anastomotic site recurrence of CD after ileo-cecal resection in CD seen on colonoscopy. C. Inflammatory stricture in CD- not ideal for endoscopic dilatation, D and E- mild or non- inflammatory fibrotic stricture - ideal for endoscopic dilatation, F. endoscopic balloon dilatation being performed in CD stricture.

than 5 aphthous lesions: i2- >5 aphthous lesions with normal mucosa between the lesions, or skip areas of larger lesions or lesions confined to the ileocolonic anastomosis (i.e., <1 cm in length); i3-diffuse aphthous ileitis with diffusely inflamed mucosa; i,4-diffuse inflammation with larger ulcers, nodules, and/or narrowing.

Apart from prediction of post operative recurrence, treatment can be decided based upon the scoring system for recurrent CD [37].

Ileo-colonoscopy is the standard test to diagnose post operative recurrence of CD (**Figure 4A, B**), but emerging data shows that VCE can diagnose CD recurrence in significantly higher number of patients compared to ileo-colonoscopy and can lead to change in management in more than half of the patients [38–40]. A recent study has shown that ileal rather than anastomotic recurrence is more likely to predict long term outcomes in CD (**Figure 4A, B**) [41]. Hence, VCE has the potential to improve clinical outcomes in postoperative CD beyond the scope of ileo-colonoscopy.

4.6 Assessment of IBD-unclassified (IBD-U)

VCE in IBD-U can detect new small bowel lesions compatible with CD in 17–70% patients. However, a normal VCE can not preclude the future evolution of new small bowel lesions suggestive of CD [42, 43]. In a study 5/25 (20%) IBD- U patients with normal VCE developed CD on follow up [44]. This is particularly important in paediatric IBD. Additional information provided by VCE can impact management in this scenario [45].

5. Enteroscopy in IBD

The drawbacks of VCE like lack of therapeutic ability, low specificity and inability to perform histological confirmation are circumvented by DAE. DAE includes double balloon enteroscopy (DBE), single balloon enteroscopy (SBE), balloon guided enteroscopy (BGE) and spiral enteroscopy. The detailed technical aspects of all DAE techniques are out of the scope of the current chapter.

5.1 SBE/DBE

SBE, in contrast to DBE does not have any balloon at the tip of the enteroscope and hence handling of the balloon control unit is easier. DBE may be preferred over SBE in the presence of adhesions. Additionally, during retrograde DAE, which is technically more difficult than antegrade DAE, SBE may be more prone to backward slippage compared to DBE due to lack of balloon at the enteroscope tip [46].

5.2 BGE

A novel through the scope (TTS), on-demand balloon assisted enteroscopy have been recently described which can be performed by push and pull technique by a disposable advancing balloon through the working channel of a colonoscope with a minimal working channel diameter of 3.7 mm. The advantage of this technique is feasibility, safety and shorter procedure duration without adverse events. The learning curve is also smaller as compared to other DAE techniques. The main drawback of this procedure is sub-optimal stability of endoscope during therapeutic procedures due to lack of aching balloon. This has been recently overcome by using a colonoscope with an integrated latex free balloon at the bending section. In a multi-centre study in adults, the average insertion length were 158 cm (50–350 cm) and 89 cm (20–150 cm) from antegrade and retrograde approach respectively, with an average procedure time of 15.5 minutes [47]. More recently, the feasibility and safety of this NaviAid AB device (Smart Medical Systems Ltd., Ra'anana, Israel) has been shown in paediatric population [48]. Therapeutic interventions can be performed after removing the balloon catheter. This novel technique obviates the need for a enteroscope and setting up of over-tube balloons.

5.3 SE/NMSE

Spiral enteroscopy(SE) involves the use of over-tube with raised spiral edges which is rotated clockwise for advancement of enteroscope pleating small bowel loops. The over-tube has been now been replaced by novel motorised spiral enteroscopy (NMSE) composed of a reusable endoscope with integrated motor permitting rotation of a short spiral over-tube in the insertion tube portion of the endoscope and a motor control unit. The motor control unit is composed of a foot pedal and visual force gauge. The advantages of NMSE are shorter procedure time, relative ease of use, high diagnostic yield (>80%), higher total enteroscopy rates (>60%) [49–51]. Therapeutic interventions like stricture dilatation and retrieval of retained capsule endoscope have been described with NMSE [52]. Due to large diameter of overture in NMSE, it is not suitable for use in children.

5.4 Indications of DAE in CD

DAE in CD is indicated particularly in suspected isolated small bowel CD in whom ileo-colonoscopy/ small bowel cross sectional imaging are inconclusive and histological diagnosis can alter patient management (**Figure 3D-F**). In patients with established CD, DAE can diagnose and treat stenotic complications (**Figure 4C-F**), assess mucosal healing for adjusting medical therapy and precisely locate lesions to direct targeted resection (**Figure 2**) [9].

DAE in suspected and established CD is done for diagnostic and therapeutic intent respectively. In suspected CD, DAE is performed to confirm CD beyond the reach of endoscopy and ileo-colonoscopy by obtaining biopsy and thus excluding alternative diagnosis like tuberculosis and small bowel malignancy. The diagnostic yield ranges between 22–70% in suspected CD.

5.4.1 Diagnostic DAE

Diagnostic yield is particularly higher if DAE is preceded by other small bowel investigations like CTE/MRE/VCE which help to identify the lesion and guide insertion route (oral or rectal). Total enteroscopy rates in this setting ranges from 20–80% [53, 54]. Diagnostic yield of DAE is comparable to VCE according to two meta-analysis which concluded that VCE should be considered first due to non-invasive nature [55, 56]. But, histological confirmation can not be obtained by VCE which is important in areas where infections (like tuberculosis) predominate. It should be borne in mind that DAE is technically challenging specially in the presence of adhesions, associated with higher rates of complications (0.72% major complications rate, 10 times higher perforation rate compared to colonoscopy) in CD and requires deep sedation/general anaesthesia [57, 58]. Perforation risk is higher in patients with active CD, altered anatomy and anastomotic ulcerations [58]. Hence, DAE should be performed only if the findings can alter therapeutic management. In a prospective study, DAE led to step up in therapy in three forth of CD patients leading to clinical remission in nearly 90% patients [59].

Most of the studies on DAE in CD patients has been done with SBE or DBE. The diagnostic yield (**Table 3**) of DAE in suspected and known CD are 27%–79% and 53%–87% respectively. The agreement between small bowel imaging and DAE is higher in patients with known CD (75.6%) compared to those with suspected CD

Author	DAE system	Patient subgroup	Study design	Suspected CD (n)	Known CD (n)	Diagnostic yield suspected CD (%)	Diagnostic yield confirmed CD (%)	Impact on management: suspected CD (%)	Impact on management: confirmed CD (%)
Broide et al, 2020	BGE	Paediatric IBD	Prospective	15 (IBD)	16 (IBD)				
Holleran et al, 2018	SBE	Adult CD	Retrospective	13	39	39	77	69	
Tun et al, 2016	DBE	Adult CD	Retrospective	100	0			45	
Christian et al, 2016	Retrograde SBE	Adult CD	Retrospective	29		41.4		17	
Rahman et al, 2015	DBE	Adult CD	Retrospective	43	38	79	87	77	82
Navaneethan et al, 2014	SBE or DBE	Adult CD	Retrospective	22	43	27	53		53
Schulz et al, 2014	DBE	Adult CD	Retrospective	16	0	69			
Urs et al, 2014	DBE	Paediatric CD	Prospective	3	5			66	100
Uchida et al,2012	DBE	Paediatric CD	Prospective	8	4			75	75
De Riddler et al, 2012	SBE	Paediatric CD	Prospective	14	6			57	83
Di Nardo, 2012	SBE	Paediatric CD	Prospective	16	14			87	64
Möschler et al, 2011	DBE	Adult CD	Prospective	193		47			
Kondo et al, 2010	DBE	Adult CD	Retrospective	25	50	47		53	

Author	DAE system	Patient subgroup	Study design	Suspected CD (n)	Known CD (n)	Diagnostic yield suspected CD (%)	Diagnostic yield confirmed CD (%)	Impact on management: suspected CD (%)	Impact on management: confirmed CD (%)
Mensink et al, 2009	DBE	Adult CD	Retrospective	0	40	60		75	

Table 3.
Summary of studies on diagnostic yield of device assisted enteroscopy (DAE) in Crohn's disease (CD); SBE- single balloon enteroscopy, DBE- double balloon enteroscopy, BGE- balloon guided enteroscopy [69–78, 81–86]

(36.4%). The diagnostic yield is higher if DAE is preceded by prior small bowel evaluation to decide the insertion route. The diagnostic yield drops drastically if DAE is performed for non-specific abdominal symptoms. DAE can significantly impact patient management in 17% to 82% [60–68].

5.4.2 Therapeutic DAE

DAE can be performed with therapeutic intent in established CD to dilate short (<5 cm), non-inflammatory strictures (4E-F), insert stents, inject intra-lesional steroid, remove foreign body like capsule or Bezoar and rarely to treat major haemorrhage in CD. Reported technical success for stricture dilatation ranges from 60–80% and perforation rates as high as 9% has been described [69].

Strictures in Crohn's disease (CD) are secondary to inflammation, fibrosis, or both. The risk of fibrotic stricture increases with the disease duration; such strictures are seen in 30% to 35% of patients within 10 years of diagnosis of CD [36]. Despite biologic use, the incidence of strictures remains unchanged in CD [70]. Endoscopic stricturotomy and balloon dilatation are the most common endoscopic procedures performed for CD strictures. However, both are associated with a high risk of recurrence, re-intervention and surgery.

The use of self-expanding metal stents (SEMS) have been reported for CD strictures with high technical success rate. However, it is associated with risk of perforation, stent migration, and fistula [71, 72]. Premature stent failure is the drawback of biodegradable stents, used to circumvent adverse events of SEMS. Currently available biodegradable stents are not specifically designed for CD strictures [73–75].

In a recent single-center series of CD patients, removable SEMS therapy for short (6 cm) fibrostenotic strictures of terminal ileum/ ileocolonic anastomoses was technically successful in 95.8%. The stents were removed within 7 days. On long-term follow-up (3–50 months), none of the patients required stricture-related surgery [76]. The global interventional inflammatory bowel disease (IBD) group recommendations has positioned fully covered SEMS for refractory strictures in selected patients failing balloon dilatation and endoscopic stricturotomy [77].

The technical success rate (defined as successful dilatation leading to endoscope passage) of endoscopic balloon dilatation (EBD) for CD strictures varies from 72% to 100% (**Table 4**). The clinical success, defined as in improvement in patient's obstructive symptoms, is around 60%.

The dilatation diameter varied from 12.4 to 17 mm with maximum of 20 mm. The recurrence rate varied from 14% to 78.5% based on duration of follow up. In studies with more than 3 years of follow up, the recurrence rates were 48% and 78.5%, respectively. Overall, most recurrences can be successfully treated with repeat balloon dilatation with a cumulative surgery free rate of 78% at 3 years. So, long term high recurrence rates and need for repeated dilatation or surgery should be kept in mind prior to EBD for CD strictures [69, 78–82].

5.4.3 DAE in paediatric patients

DAE is safe and effective for children aged >3 years and weight > 14 kg. DAE is challenging in children due to small abdominal cavity, thinner small bowel wall and a narrow lumen requiring considerable expertise. Five studies (2 SBE, 2 DBE and 1 BGE) have evaluated the role of DAE in paediatric IBD. In these studies, DAE either led to treatment escalation or was used to perform stricture dilatation. Definitive IBD type was ascertained in patients with IBD-U after BGE in a feasibility and safety study. These studies did not report any major complications with diagnostic or therapeutic DAE. DAE related complications in paediatric patients are reported

Author	DAE system	Study design	CD (n)	Total number of dilations (per patient mean)	Dilation diameter: mean (range) (mm)	Technical success (%)	Clinical success (%)	Perforation (%)	Follow up (months)	Recurrence rate (%)
Hirai et al, 2018	SBE or DBE	Prospective	95	90 (1)	15 (8–20)	94	70	0	24	NA
Holleran et al, 2018	SBE	Retrospective	13	14 (1)	13 (12–15)	100	80	0	8	23
Sunada et al, 2016	DBE	Retrospective	85	321 (3.8)	12.4 (8–20)		87	5	41.9 (0–141)	78.5
Navaneethan et al, 2014	SBE or DBE	Retrospective	6	7 (1.16)	43	100	100	16		
Hirai et al, 2014	DBE	Retrospective	65		NA [12–18]	80	80	1.5		48
Gill et al, 2014	DBE	Retrospective	10	17 (1.8)	13.5 (10–16.5)	80	70	20		14
Hirai et al,2010	DBE	Retrospective	25	55 (2.2)	NA [12–18]	72	72	0	11	22
Kondo et al, 2010	DBE	Retrospective	8	18 (1.5)		100	87.5	0		
Despott et al, 2009	DBE	Prospective	11	18 (2)	15.4 (12–20)	73	73	9	20.5	25
Ohmiya et al, 2009	DBE	Retrospective	16	NA	NA [8–20]	96	69	0	16	31
Pohl et al, 2007	Push enteroscopy	R	16	15 (1.5)	17 (12–20)	80	60	0	10	40
Fukumoto et al, 2007	DBE	Prospective	193	35 (1.52)	NA	NA	74	0	12	26

Table 4.
Summary of studies on endoscopic balloon dilatation of Crohn's disease small bowel strictures with device assisted enteroscopy (DAE); SBE- single balloon enteroscopy, DBE- double balloon enteroscopy, BGE- balloon guided enteroscopy [78–82].

mostly with therapeutic DAE. Overall complications with a large DBE series (n = 257) is 5.4% (10.4% in patients <10 years). The largest SBE series (n = 189) does not report any major adverse events except for transient pain and distension (28%) and one case of self limited bleeding [48, 73, 81–87].

5.4.4 Complications of DAE

Major complications like bleeding, perforation or pancreatitis with DAE are found in about 0.72% (which may be higher in patients with Crohn's disease). Rate of perforation with DAE is around 0.11% according to results of a large Japanese registry of nearly thirty thousand patients. The risk of perforation was nine fold higher in IBD patients on steroids [88]. The rate of perforation with endoscopic balloon dilatation can be as high as 9% [60]. Bleeding after DAE has been reported in around 2.5% which is mostly self limiting [61]. Pancreatitis can occur in upto 0.3% patients after DAE from antegrade approach [89]. In paediatric IBD settings, although overall complication rates Of upto 5.4% is reported, none reported major complications even with therapeutic procedures [75].

6. Intra-operative enteroscopy in CD

Earlier studies have shown that IOE has useful role in surgical decision making in ulcers and strictures in CD [90, 91]. In our experience (unpublished observation), IOE helped to identify ulcers/strictures missed on initial pre-operative evaluation (31.8%, 7/22) (**Figure 1D**). In case of multiple strictures, IOE also helped in deciding the extent of surgical resection. In 30% (6/20) of the cases, strictures were severe (not allowing enteroscope passage) and rest had mild, passable strictures. Of the subjects with severe strictures (6/20), 3 were judged to have mild stricture on inspection and palpation during laparotomy. Hence, IOE has important role in guiding surgical management of small intestinal ulcers/strictures [82, 83].

7. Conclusion

Small bowel endoscopy is essential for both diagnostic and therapeutic purposes in suspected and confirmed CD. This is particularly valuable for diagnosis when upper endoscopy, ileo-colonoscopy and cross sectional small bowel imaging are non-contributory or non-diagnostic. VCE is useful if there are no obstructive symptoms or known stenosis although DAE guided biopsy is important in scenarios when alternative pathology requires exclusion specially in countries where tuberculosis is endemic. Newer devices like motorised spiral enteroscopy and balloon guided enteroscopy have revolutionised the management of small bowel CD. DAE is be safe and effective in both adults and children with CD. Apart from therapeutic interventions like foreign body retrieval, endoscopic balloon dilatation, stent placement and haemostasis; small bowel endoscopy could be useful in postoperative CD recurrence detection and document mucosal healing and response to therapy.

Conflicts of interest

None.

Financial disclosures

None.

Author details

Partha Pal, D. Nageshwar Reddy and Zaheer Nabi*
Asian Institute of Gastroenterology Hyderabad, Telangana, India

*Address all correspondence to: zaheernabi1978@gmail.com

IntechOpen

© 2021 The Author(s). Licensee IntechOpen. This chapter is distributed under the terms of the Creative Commons Attribution License (http://creativecommons.org/licenses/by/3.0), which permits unrestricted use, distribution, and reproduction in any medium, provided the original work is properly cited.

References

[1] Kim M, Jang HJ. The role of small bowel endoscopy in small bowel Crohn's disease: when and how? Intest Res. 2016 Jul;14(3):211-7. doi: 10.5217/ir.2016.14.3.211. Epub 2016 Jun 27. PMID: 27433142; PMCID: PMC4945524.

[2] Pennazio M, Spada C, Eliakim R, et al. Small-bowel capsule endoscopy and device-assisted enteroscopy for diagnosis and treatment of small-bowel disorders: European Society of Gastrointestinal Endoscopy (ESGE) Clinical Guideline. Endoscopy. 2015 Apr;47(4):352-76.

[3] van Assche G, Dignass A, Panes J et al. The second European evidence-based Consensus on the diagnosis and management of Crohn's dis- ease: Definitions and diagnosis. J Crohns Colitis 2010; 4: 7-27

[4] Jensen MD, Nathan T, Rafaelsen SR et al. Ileoscopy reduces the need for small bowel imaging in suspected Crohn's disease. Dan Med J 2012; 59: A4491

[5] Bourreille A, Ignjatovic A, Aabakken L, et al., World Organisation of Digestive Endoscopy (OMED) and the European Crohn's and Colitis Organisation (ECCO). Role of small-bowel endoscopy in the management of patients with inflammatory bowel disease: an international OMED-ECCO consensus. Endoscopy 2009; 41:618-637.

[6] Condino G, Calabrese E, Onali S et al. Small bowel capsule endoscopy for assessing early postoperative recurrence of Crohn's disease: a pro- spective longitudinal study. Gastroenterol 2013; 144 Suppl 1: S425

[7] Mehdizadeh S, Chen G, Enayati PJ et al. Diagnostic yield of capsule en- doscopy in ulcerative colitis and inflammatory bowel disease of un-classified type (IBDU). Endoscopy 2008; 40: 30-35

[8] Shen B, Remzi FH, Santisi J et al. Application of wireless capsule endos- copy for the evaluation of iron deficiency anemia in patients with ileal pouches. J Clin Gastroenterol 2008; 42: 897-902

[9] Maaser C, Sturm A, Vavricka SR, et al; European Crohn's and Colitis Organisation [ECCO] and the European Society of Gastrointestinal and Abdominal Radiology [ESGAR]. ECCO-ESGAR Guideline for Diagnostic Assessment in IBD Part 1: Initial diagnosis, monitoring of known IBD, detection of complications. J Crohns Colitis. 2019 Feb 1;13(2):144-164.

[10] Lashner B.Clinical features, laboratory findings, and course of Crohn's disease. In: Kirsner JV (ed) Inflammatory bowel disease. 5th edn. Philadelphia: Saunders, 2000: 305-314

[11] Banerjee R, Pal P, Mak JWY, Ng SC. Challenges in the diagnosis and management of inflammatory bowel disease in resource-limited settings in Asia. Lancet Gastroenterol Hepatol. 2020 Dec;5(12):1076-1088. doi: 10.1016/S2468-1253(20)30299-5. PMID: 33181087

[12] Hilmi I, Kobayashi T. Capsule endoscopy in inflammatory bowel disease: when and how. Intest Res. 2020 Jul;18(3):265-274. doi: 10.5217/ir.2019.09165. Epub 2020 Jul 7. PMID: 32623876; PMCID: PMC7385570.

[13] Tukey M, Pleskow D, Legnani P, Cheifetz AS, Moss AC. The utility of capsule endoscopy in patients with suspected Crohn's disease. Am J Gastroenterol. 2009 Nov;104(11):2734-9. doi: 10.1038/ajg.2009.404. Epub 2009 Jul 7. PMID: 19584828

[14] Monteiro S, Boal Carvalho P, Dias de Castro F, et al. Capsule endoscopy: diagnostic accuracy of Lewis score in patients with suspected Crohn's disease. Inflamm Bowel Dis 2015; 21:2241-2246.

[15] Chateau T, Damico F, Zallot C, Mathieu N, Peyrin-Biroulet L. Crohn's Disease Only Visible on Small Bowel Capsule Endoscopy: A New Entity. Dig Dis Sci. 2020 Aug 18. doi: 10.1007/s10620-020-06553-3. Epub ahead of print. Erratum in: Dig Dis Sci. 2020 Sep 25;: PMID: 32809105.

[16] Liao Z, Gao R, Xu C et al. Indications and detection, completion, and retention rates of small-bowel capsule endoscopy: a systematic review. Gastrointest Endosc 2010; 71: 280-286

[17] Yadav A, Heigh RI, Hara AK, et al. Performance of the patency capsule compared with nonenteroclysis radiologic examinations in patients with known or suspected intestinal strictures. Gastrointest Endosc. 2011 Oct;74(4):834-9.

[18] Dionisio PM, Gurudu SR, Leighton JA et al. Capsule endoscopy has a significantly higher diagnostic yield in patients with suspected and established small-bowel Crohn's disease: a meta-analysis. Am J Gastro- enterol 2010; 105: 1240-1248

[19] Dussault C, Gower-Rousseau C, Salleron J, Vernier-Massouille G, Branche J, Colombel JF, Maunoury V. Small bowel capsule endoscopy for management of Crohn's disease: a retrospective tertiary care centre experience. Dig Liver Dis. 2013 Jul;45(7):558-61. doi: 10.1016/j.dld.2012.11.004. Epub 2012 Dec 11. PMID: 23238033.

[20] Kopylov U, Nemeth A, Koulaouzidis A, et al. Small bowel capsule endoscopy in the management of established Crohn's disease: clinical impact, safety, and correlation with inflammatory biomarkers. Inflamm Bowel Dis. 2015 Jan;21(1):93-100.

[21] Ben-Horin S, Lahat A, Amitai MM,et al; Israeli IBD Research Nucleus (IIRN). Assessment of small bowel mucosal healing by video capsule endoscopy for the prediction of short-term and long-term risk of Crohn's disease flare: a prospective cohort study. Lancet Gastroenterol Hepatol. 2019 Jul;4(7):519-528. doi: 10.1016/S2468-1253(19)30088-3. Epub 2019 May 9. PMID: 31080097.

[22] Oliva S, Aloi M, Viola F, Mallardo S, Civitelli F, Maccioni F, Hassan C, Papoff P, Cucchiara S, Cohen SA. A Treat to Target Strategy Using Panenteric Capsule Endoscopy in Pediatric Patients With Crohn's Disease. Clin Gastroenterol Hepatol. 2019 Sep;17(10):2060-2067.e1. doi: 10.1016/j.cgh.2018.10.015. Epub 2018 Oct 13. PMID: 30326301.

[23] Cheon JH, Kim YS, Lee IS et al. Can we predict spontaneous capsule passage after retention? A nationwide study to evaluate the incidence and clinical outcomes of capsule retention Endoscopy 2007; 39: 1046-1052

[24] Viazis N, Zacharakis G, Saprikis E et al. A single center experience of 2300 consecutive patients undergoing capsule endoscopy: indications and diagnostic yield. Endoscopy 2011; 43: A129

[25] Mow WS, Lo SK, Targan SR et al. Initial experience with wireless capsule enteroscopy in the diagnosis and management of inflammatory bowel disease. Clin Gastroenterol Hepatol 2004; 2: 31-40

[26] Gralnek IM, de Franchis R, Seidman E et al. Development of a capsule endoscopy scoring index for small bowel mucosal inflammatory change. Aliment Pharmacol Ther 2008; 27: 146-154

[27] Gal E, Geller A, Fraser G et al. Assessment and validation of the new

capsule endoscopy Crohn's disease activity index (CECDAI). Dig Dis Sci 2008; 53: 1933-1937

[28] Omori T, Kambayashi H, Murasugi S, Ito A, Yonezawa M, Nakamura S, Tokushige K. Comparison of Lewis Score and Capsule Endoscopy Crohn's Disease Activity Index in Patients with Crohn's Disease. Dig Dis Sci. 2020 Apr;65(4):1180-1188. doi: 10.1007/s10620-019-05837-7. Epub 2019 Sep 20. PMID: 31541367.

[29] Yablecovitch D, Lahat A, Neuman S, et al. The Lewis score or the capsule endoscopy Crohn's disease activity index: which one is better for the assessment of small bowel inflammation in established Crohn's disease? Therap Adv Gastroenterol 2018;11:1756283X17747780.

[30] Dussault C, Gower-Rousseau C, Salleron J, Vernier-Massouille G, Branche J, Colombel JF, Maunoury V. Small bowel capsule endoscopy for management of Crohn's disease: a retrospective tertiary care centre experience. Dig Liver Dis. 2013 Jul;45(7):558-61. doi: 10.1016/j.dld.2012.11.004. Epub 2012 Dec 11. PMID: 23238033.

[31] Nemeth A, Kopylov U, Koulaouzidis A, Wurm Johansson G, Thorlacius H, Amre D, Eliakim R, Seidman EG, Toth E. Use of patency capsule in patients with established Crohn's disease. Endoscopy. 2016 Apr;48(4):373-9. doi: 10.1055/s-0034-1393560. Epub 2015 Nov 12. PMID: 26561918

[32] Spada C, Spera G, Riccioni M, Biancone L, Petruzziello L, Tringali A, Familiari P, Marchese M, Onder G, Mutignani M, Perri V, Petruzziello C, Pallone F, Costamagna G. A novel diagnostic tool for detecting functional patency of the small bowel: the Given patency capsule. Endoscopy. 2005 Sep;37(9):793-800. doi: 10.1055/s-2005-870246. PMID: 16116528.

[33] Caunedo-Alvarez A, Romero-Vazquez J, Herrerias-Gutierrez JM. Patency and Agile capsules. World J Gastroenterol 2008; 14: 5269-5273.

[34] Rasmussen B, Nathan T, Jensen MD. Symptomatic patency capsule retention in suspected Crohn's disease. J Crohns Colitis 2016; 10: 1445-1447.

[35] Garg S, Anand R, Dubin E, Kantsevoy S, Dutta S. Endoscopic management of retained patency capsules. Endoscopy 2014; 46: Suppl 1 UCTN:E662-3.

[36] Cosnes J, Cattan S, Blain A, et al. Long-term evolution of disease behavior of Crohn's disease. Inflamm Bowel Dis 2002;8:244-50.

[37] Rutgeerts P, Geboes K, Vantrappen G, Beyls J, Kerremans R, Hiele M. Predictability of the postoperative course of Crohn's disease. Gastroenterology 1990;99:956-963.

[38] Pons Beltrán V, Nos P, Bastida G, et al. Evaluation of postsurgi- cal recurrence in Crohn's disease: a new indication for cap- sule endoscopy? Gastrointest Endosc 2007;66:533-540.

[39] Bourreille A, Jarry M, D'Halluin PN, et al. Wireless capsule endoscopy versus ileocolonoscopy for the diagnosis of postop- erative recurrence of Crohn's disease: a prospective study. Gut 2006;55:978-983.

[40] Sorrentino D, Nguyen VQ. Clinically significant small bowel Crohn's disease might only be detected by capsule endosco- py. Inflamm Bowel Dis 2018;24:1566-1574.

[41] Hammoudi N, Auzolle C, Tran Minh ML, et al. Postoperative Endoscopic Recurrence on the

Neoterminal Ileum But Not on the Anastomosis Is Mainly Driving Long-Term Outcomes in Crohn's Disease. Am J Gastroenterol. 2020 Jul;115(7):1084-1093.

[42] Kalla R, McAlindon ME, Drew K et al. Clinical utility of capsule endoscopy in patients with Crohn's disease and inflammatory bowel disease unclassified. Eur J Gastroenterol Hepatol 2013; 25: 706-713

[43] Joossens S, Reinisch W, Vermeire S et al. The value of serologic markers in indeterminate colitis: a prospective follow-up study. Gastroenterology 2002; 122: 1242-1247

[44] Maunoury V, Sovoye G, Bourreille A et al. Value of wireless capsule endoscopy in patients with indeterminate colitis (inflammatory bowel disease type unclassified). Inflamm Bowel Dis 2007; 13: 152-155

[45] Min SB, Le-Carlson M, Singh N, et al. Video capsule endoscopy impacts decision making in pediatric IBD: a single tertiary care center experience. Inflamm Bowel Dis. 2013 Sep;19(10):2139-45.

[46] Nardo GD, Esposito G, Ziparo C, Micheli F, Masoni L, Villa MP, Parisi P, Manca MB, Baccini F, Corleto VD. Enteroscopy in children and adults with inflammatory bowel disease. World J Gastroenterol. 2020 Oct 21;26(39):5944-5958. doi: 10.3748/wjg.v26.i39.5944. PMID: 33132646; PMCID: PMC7584063.

[47] Ali R, Wild D, Shieh F, et al. Deep enteroscopy with a conventional colonoscope: initial multicenter study by using a through-the- scope balloon catheter system. Gastrointest Endosc 2015;82: 855-60.

[48] Broide E, Shalem T, Richter V, Matalon S, Shirin H. The Safety and Feasibility of a New Through-the-scope Balloon-assisted Enteroscopy in Children. J Pediatr Gastroenterol Nutr. 2020 Jul;71(1):e6-e11. doi: 10.1097/MPG.0000000000002706. PMID: 32187142.

[49] Ramchandani M, Rughwani H, Inavolu P, et al. Diagnostic yield and therapeutic impact of novel motorized spiral enteroscopy in small-bowel disorders: a single-center, real-world experience from a tertiary care hospital (with video). Gastrointest Endosc. 2020 Jul 12:S0016-5107(20)34541-7. doi: 10.1016/j.gie.2020.07.001. Epub ahead of print. PMID: 32663489.

[50] Beyna T, Arvanitakis M, Schneider M, et al. Total motorized spiral enteroscopy: first prospective clinical feasibility trial. Gastrointest Endosc. 2020 Oct 31:S0016-5107(20)34934-8. doi: 10.1016/j.gie.2020.10.028. Epub ahead of print. PMID: 33144239.

[51] Beyna T, Arvanitakis M, Schneider M, et al. Motorised spiral enteroscopy: first prospective clinical feasibility study. Gut. 2020 Apr 24:gutjnl-2019-319908. doi: 10.1136/gutjnl-2019-319908. Epub ahead of print. PMID: 32332141.

[52] Inavolu P, Singh AP, Kanakagiri H, Reddy DN, Ramchandani M. Motorized spiral enteroscope-assisted retrieval of video capsule in a patient with Crohn's disease. VideoGIE. 2020 Jul 22;5(10):488-491. doi: 10.1016/j.vgie.2020.05.014. PMID: 33103006; PMCID: PMC7570370.

[53] Gay G, Delvaux M. Double balloon enteroscopy in Crohn's disease and related disorders: our experience. Gastrointest Endosc 2007; 66: S82 – S90

[54] Manes G, Imbesi V, Ardizzone S et al. Use of double-balloon enteroscopy in the management of patients with Crohn's disease: feasibility and diagnostic yield in a high-volume centre

for inflammatory bowel disease. Surg Endosc 2009; 23: 2790-2795

[55] Pasha SF, Leighton JA, Das A et al. Double-balloon enteroscopy and capsule endoscopy have comparable diagnostic yield in small-bowel disease: a meta-analysis. Clin Gastroenterol Hepatol 2008; 6: 671-676

[56] Chen X, Ran ZH, Tong JL. A meta-analysis of the yield of capsule endoscopy compared to double-balloon enteroscopy in patients with small bowel diseases. World J Gastroenterol 2007; 13: 4372-4378

[57] Xin L, Liao Z, Jiang YP et al. Indications, detectability, positive findings, total enteroscopy, and complications of diagnostic double-balloon endoscopy: a systematic review of data over the first decade of use. Gastrointest Endosc 2011; 74: 563-570

[58] Gerson L, Chiorean M, Tokar J et al. Complications associated with double balloon enteroscopy: the US experience. Am J Gastroenterol 2008; 103: S109 – S110

[59] Mensink PB, Aktas H, Zelinkova Z et al. Impact of double-balloon enteroscopy findings on the management of Crohn's disease. Scand J Gastroenterol 2010; 45: 483-489

[60] Navaneethan U, Vargo JJ, Menon KV, Sanaka MR, Tsai CJ. Impact of balloon-assisted enteroscopy on the diagnosis and management of suspected and established small-bowel Crohn's disease. Endosc Int Open 2014; 2: E201-E206

[61] Rahman A, Ross A, Leighton JA, et al. Double- balloon enteroscopy in Crohn's disease: findings and impact on management in a multicenter retrospective study. Gastrointest Endosc 2015; 82: 102-107 [PMID: 25840927 DOI: 10.1016/j.gie.2014.12.039]

[62] Tun GS, Rattehalli D, Sanders DS, McAlindon ME, Drew K, Sidhu R. Clinical utility of double-balloon enteroscopy in suspected Crohn's disease: a single-centre experience. Eur J Gastroenterol Hepatol 2016; 28: 820-825

[63] Holleran G, Valerii G, Tortora A, et al. The use of single balloon enteroscopy in Crohn's disease and its impact on clinical outcome. Scand J Gastroenterol 2018; 53: 925-929 [PMID: 29966446 DOI: 10.1080/00365521.2018.1476914]

[64] Di Nardo G, Oliva S, Aloi M, et al. Usefulness of single-balloon enteroscopy in pediatric Crohn's disease. Gastrointest Endosc 2012; 75: 80-86

[65] Kondo J, Iijima H, Abe T, et al. Roles of double-balloon endoscopy in the diagnosis and treatment of Crohn's disease: a multicenter experience. J Gastroenterol 2010; 45: 713-720

[66] Möschler O, May A, Müller MK, Ell C; German DBE Study Group. Complications in and performance of double-balloon enteroscopy (DBE): results from a large prospective DBE database in Germany. Endoscopy 2011; 43: 484-489

[67] Christian KE, Kapoor K, Goldberg EM. Performance characteristics of retrograde single-balloon endoscopy: A single center experience. World J Gastrointest Endosc 2016; 8: 501-507

[68] Mensink PB, Groenen MJ, van Buuren HR, Kuipers EJ, van der Woude CJ. Double-balloon enteroscopy in Crohn's disease patients suspected of small bowel activity: findings and clinical impact. J Gastroenterol 2009; 44: 271-276

[69] Despott EJ, Gupta A, Burling D et al. Effective dilation of small-bowel strictures by double-balloon enteroscopy in patients with

symptomatic Crohn's disease (with video). Gastrointest Endosc 2009; 70: 1030-1036

[70] Rieder F, Zimmermann EM, Remzi FH, et al. Crohn's disease complicated by strictures: a systematic review. Gut 2013;62:1072-84.

[71] Navaneethan U, Lourdusamy V, Njei B, et al. Endoscopic balloon dilation in the management of strictures in Crohn's disease: a systematic review and meta-analysis of nonrandomized trials. Surg Endosc 2016;30:5434-43.

[72] Lan N, Shen B. Endoscopic stricturotomy with needle knife in the treatment of strictures from inflammatory bowel disease. Inflamm Bowel Dis 2017;23:502-13.

[73] Loras C, Pérez-Roldan F, Gornals JB, et al. Endoscopic treatment with self-expanding metal stents for Crohn's disease strictures. Aliment Pharmacol Ther 2012;36:833-9.

[74] Attar A, Branche J, Coron E, et al. P608 New anti-migration extractible metal stents for Crohn's disease strictures: a nationwide GETAID-SFED cohort study. J Crohns Colitis 2017;11:S389-90.

[75] Karstensen JG. Biodegradable stents for the treatment of bowel strictures in Crohn's disease: technical results and challenges. Endosc Int Open 2016:E296-300.

[76] Das R, Singh R, Din S, et al. Therapeutic resolution of focal, predominantly anastomotic Crohn's disease strictures using removable stents: outcomes from a single-center case series in the United Kingdom. Gastrointest Endosc 2020;92:344-52.

[77] Shen B, Kochhar G, Navaneethan U, et al. Practical guidelines on endoscopic treatment for Crohn's disease strictures: a consensus statement from the Global Interventional Inflammatory Bowel Disease Group. Lancet Gastroenterol Hepatol 2020;5:393-405.

[78] Hirai F, Beppu T, Sou S, Seki T, Yao K, Matsui T. Endoscopic balloon dilatation using double-balloon endoscopy is a useful and safe treatment for small intestinal strictures in Crohn's disease. Dig Endosc 2010; 22: 200-204

[79] Gill RS, Kaffes AJ. Small bowel stricture characterization and outcomes of dilatation by double-balloon enteroscopy: a single-centre experience. Therap Adv Gastroenterol 2014; 7: 108-114

[80] Hirai F, Beppu T, Takatsu N, et al. Long-term outcome of endoscopic balloon dilation for small bowel strictures in patients with Crohn's disease. Dig Endosc 2014; 26: 545-551

[81] Sunada K, Shinozaki S, Nagayama M, et al. Long-term Outcomes in Patients with Small Intestinal Strictures Secondary to Crohn's Disease After Double-balloon Endoscopy-assisted Balloon Dilation. Inflamm Bowel Dis 2016; 22:380-386

[82] Hirai F, Andoh A, Ueno F, et al. Efficacy of Endoscopic Balloon Dilation for Small Bowel Strictures in Patients With Crohn's Disease: A Nationwide, Multi-centre, Open-label, Prospective Cohort Study. J Crohns Colitis 2018; 12: 394-401

[83] Yokoyama K, Yano T, Kumagai H, Mizuta K, Ono S, Imagawa T, Yamamoto H, Yamagata T. Double-balloon Enteroscopy for Pediatric Patients: Evaluation of Safety and Efficacy in 257 Cases. J Pediatr Gastroenterol Nutr 2016; 63: 34-40

[84] de Ridder L, Mensink PB, Lequin MH, Aktas H, de Krijger RR, van der Woude CJ, Escher JC. Single- balloon enteroscopy, magnetic resonance enterography, and abdominal US useful

for evaluation of small- bowel disease in children with (suspected) Crohn's disease. Gastrointest Endosc 2012; 75: 87-94

[85] Urs AN, Martinelli M, Rao P, Thomson MA. Diagnostic and therapeutic utility of double-balloon enteroscopy in children. J Pediatr Gastroenterol Nutr 2014; 58: 204-212

[86] Uchida K, Yoshiyama S, Inoue M, Koike Y, Yasuda H, Fujikawa H, Okita Y, Araki T, Tanaka K, Kusunoki M. Double balloon enteroscopy for pediatric inflammatory bowel disease. Pediatr Int 2012; 54: 806-809

[87] Reddy PM, Kulkarni S, Nabi Z, et al. Single balloon enteroscopy in children for evaluation of small bowel diseases in children: A large, tertiary center study. J Pediatr Surg. 2020 Nov 2:S0022-3468(20)30778-8. doi: 10.1016/j.jpedsurg.2020.10.025. Epub ahead of print. PMID: 33189296

[88] Odagiri H, Matsui H, Fushimi K, Kaise M, Yasunaga H. Factors associated with perforation related to diagnostic balloon-assisted enteroscopy: analysis of a national inpatient database in Japan. Endoscopy 2015; 47: 143-146

[89] Gerson LB, Tokar J, Chiorean M, et al. Complications associated with double balloon enteroscopy at nine US centers. Clin Gastroenterol Hepatol 2009; 7: 1177-1182, 1182.e1-1182. e3

[90] Hotokezaka M, Jimi SI, Hidaka H, et al. Role of intraoperative enteroscopy for surgical decision making with Crohn's disease. Surg Endosc. 2007;21(7):1238-1242. doi:10.1007/s00464-006-9154-z

[91] Esaki M, Matsumoto T, Hizawa K, et al. Intraoperative enteroscopy detects more lesions but is not predictive of postoperative recurrence in Crohn's disease. Surg Endosc. 2001;15(5):455-459. doi:10.1007/s004640000174

Section 4

Endoscopic Ultrasound

Chapter 5

Endoscopic Ultrasound Assessment of the Duodenal Wall Lesions

Andrada Seicean, Voicu Rednic and Radu Seicean

Abstract

Subepithelial tumors (SETs) in the upper digestive tract are rare and only 10% of are located in the duodenum. Assessment of lesions protruding from the duodenal wall is difficult. Upper gastrointestinal (GI) endoscopy and computed tomography (CT) are not able to completely distinguish between different tumors and guide their subsequent management. Endoscopic ultrasonography (EUS) has a significant diagnostic yield in this context. EUS is able to accurately diagnose duodenal lesions, perform a biopsy if considered useful, guide the approach for resection and provide appropriate follow-up. SETs reported during upper GI endoscopy are more commonly cysts, polyps, lipomas, Brunner's gland adenoma, ectopic pancreas, gastrointestinal stromal tumors (GISTs) or neuroendocrine tumors (NETs). In addition, although more rarely, adenocarcinomas and lymphomas can be identified. EUS should be performed for any duodenal lesion larger than 1 cm that lacks the endoscopic characteristics of a cyst or a lipoma.

Keywords: subepithelial tumors, intramural lesions, endoscopic ultrasound, duodenum, endoscopy, interventional endoscopy

1. Introduction

Lesions of the upper gastrointestinal (GI) tract are usually assessed by esophagogastroduodenoscopy (EGD), but less importance is shown for lesions of the small intestine. Protrusive lesions of the small intestine can arise from mucosa, with endoscopic features that allow their characterization. However, deep organ involvement cannot be assessed by endoscopy. The same is true for lesions from subepithelial layers, known as subepithelial lesions (SELs). These appear as bulging lesions covered by normal mucosa, and are firm as they are "palpated" with closed biopsy forceps. The mucosa covering these lesions is usually normal, and standard biopsies or "bite-to-bite" biopsies have low diagnostic accuracy. Assessing these lesions can be difficult, as computed tomography (CT) and magnetic resonance imaging (MRI) lack the resolution to properly describe them because of their size.

Endoscopic ultrasound (EUS) overcomes these drawbacks. Due to high resolution and ability to differentiate between all layers of the GI tract [1], EUS assesses the layer of origin, size, morphologic features, and involvement of the neighboring organs. Combined with the possibility of targeted biopsies from the deeper layers, EUS is the most effective for evaluating SETs of the duodenum.

 IntechOpen

SETs of the duodenum can be true intramural lesions of the duodenal wall or extrinsic compressions. Extrinsic compression comes from adjacent structures, like the gallbladder or blood vessels. Around 1 in 5 SETs found in the upper GI tract is an extramural compression [2, 3]. Data regarding external compressions on the duodenum are few, but clinical experience suggests that they are less frequent than in the stomach. Intramural lesions can be true submucosal or pseudo-submucosal lesions. The latter are usually polyps or inflammatory lesions. True submucosal lesions originate from one of the deeper layers of the duodenal wall. Benign SETs of the duodenum include cysts, gastrointestinal stromal tumors (GISTs), leiomyomas (very rare) of the minor papilla (which at EGD can be confused with SETs), lipomas, neuroendocrine tumors (NETs) and ectopic pancreas. Malignant SETs can be malignant mesenchymal tumors, adenocarcinomas or lymphomas (**Table 1**).

A correct and complete diagnosis of an SET, including extension and proximity to other structures, is essential in deciding the following steps, as the complex localization and surroundings of the duodenum make surgical interventions difficult. Its thin walls and proximity to the biliary and pancreatic ducts makes even endoscopic therapeutic interventions more prone to serious complications like perforation. In this context, the diagnosis, prognosis and possible therapeutic options should always be properly weighed and presented to the patient before a decision is made.

SETs should be resected, endoscopically or surgically, if there is a suspicion of malignancy or if they are symptomatic. Tumors with malignant potential, like GISTs or NETs, should be resected, or in certain circumstances followed endoscopically. EUS can help guide the treatment. Generally, lesions limited to the mucosa and submucosa can be removed endoscopically, with a high safety profile, using advanced techniques like endoscopic submucosal resection (ESD). Tumors arising from the muscularis usually need surgical intervention.

	Xu et al. [4]	**Markovic et al. [5]**	**Kawamoto et al. [6]**
Total number	169	80	24
Mucosal lesions			
Inflammatory protruding or polyps	36 (21%)	13 (16%)	1(4%)
Submucosal lesions			
Cysts	40 (24%)	—	8(34%)
Brunner's adenoma	25(15%)	7 (9%)	6(25%)
Lymphangioma	—	—	1(4%)
Lipoma	6 (4%)	6 (8%)	1(4%)
Ectopic pancreas	19(11%)	—	1(4%)
Stromal tumors	17 (10%)	33 (41%)	1(4%)
NET	—	3 (4%)	—
Gangliocytic paraganglionas	—	—	1(4%)
Others			
Extrinsic compression	12(7%)	—	—
Minor papilla	12(7%)	—	—
Malignant tumors			
Malignant tumors	2 (1%)	18 (22%)	4(17%)

Table 1.
Different studies evaluating the final diagnosis in duodenal lesions referred to EUS. Most, but not all, are confirmed histologically after EUS.

2. Evaluation of a duodenal subepithelial tumor

2.1 Initial evaluation

SETs identified in the upper GI tract are rare, being found in around 1 in 300 EGDs [7]. Only around 10% of those are located in the duodenum [8]. The true prevalence probably remains unknown, as most SETs are asymptomatic and are found to be completely unrelated to the reason the EGD was performed. In a study involving 346 EUS examinations of upper GI SETs, 87% of the lesions were unrelated to the presenting symptoms of the patient [2]. The rare symptomatic cases usually manifest through occult bleeding or abdominal pain. Evaluation of a duodenal SET starts during the initial EGD. Its location, size, mobility and color should be noted. Modifications of the mucosa and "tenting" sign are also important. A firm lesion with a "pillow" sign is usually a lipoma, while a firm and translucent lesion can be a cyst. A central depression along mucosal irregularities can suggest an ectopic pancreas, while a central ulceration can be a sign of a GIST. Mucosal biopsies are rarely useful, as they only touch the mucosa and are unable to retrieve tissue from the lesion. More invasive methods, like "buttonhole" biopsies or jumbo forceps, are not always successful and carry high risk of adverse events [9]. If the lesion is not a cyst or lipoma, tissue acquisition should be performed for diagnosis, especially because some of the duodenal SELs have malignant potential.

2.2 Endoscopic ultrasound

The endosonographic morphology of SETs is based on size, layer of origin, echogenicity, echotexture, vascularity and lymph nodes [2]. The procedure is difficult in cases of large lesions or inaccessible regions like the jejunum, ileum or, sometimes, the fourth part of the duodenum.

Size should be reported in two orthogonal planes. There are five layers visible when examining the digestive tract. The first layer (hyperechoic) is the interface of the superficial mucosa with the contrast medium. The second layer (hypoechoic) is the deep part of the mucosa, containing the muscularis mucosae and lamina propria. The third layer (hyperechoic) is the submucosa and the interface between the submucosa and the muscularis propria. The fourth layer (hypoechoic) is the muscularis propria. The fifth layer is the serosa and the interface with adjacent structures. In addition, an SET described at EGD, as mentioned before, can actually be an extrinsic compression, originating beyond all layers. The relation with adjacent layers and structures has to be described. Are the layers immediately above and below distinguishable? Do they present ulcerations or irregularities? Can the neighboring structures be clearly distinguished or is there invasion? All these questions should be answered in a correctly redacted EUS result. The echogenicity of the tumor has to be noted. It can be anechoic (compare to the water in the lumen), hypoechoic (compare to muscularis propria), hyperechoic (compare to submucosa). The texture can also give useful information, as inhomogeneous lesions can raise suspicions of malignancy, as can irregular margins. For further description one can also mention the adjacent vascularization, presence of regional lymph nodes, hepatic lesions or free liquid in the peritoneum. Of all the characteristics mentioned, the most important are layer of origin and echogenicity (**Table 2**).

EUS without histological examination has a high diagnostic yield in duodenal SETs. Xu et al. reported an efficiency of up to 93.3% in a group of 75 duodenal SETs that had a later histological diagnosis [4]. However, diagnostic efficiency seems to be size related, as Brugge et al. reported a correct diagnosis in 45% of gastric lesions less than 2 cm in size and proposed, naturally, EUS with fine-needle aspiration (EUS-FNA) as the gold

	Layer of origin	Echogenicity	Size (mm)	Border	Malignancy potential
Duplication cysts	3rd/ external	Anechoic, without Doppler signal	—	Sharp, sometimes with five layers	No
Varices	3rd	Anechoic, with Doppler signal	—	Sharp, serpiginous shape	No
Lym phangiomas	3rd	Anechoic with internal septa, without Doppler signal	—	Sharp	No
Inflammatory fibroid polyp	2nd, 3rd	Hypoechoic, homogenous, polypoid	8–18	Indistinct	No
Neuroendocrine tumors	2nd, 3rd	Hypoechoic/ Intermediate echogenicity/ hyperechoic		Sharp	Yes
Ectopic pancreas	3rd, 4th	Hypoechoic, heterogeneous echotexture, with cysts or ducts inside, umbilication	< 5–20	Indistinct	No
GIST	2nd/4th	Hypoechoic, heterogenous, hypervascular	Any	Sharp when benign	Yes, when >30 mm, with cystic space or echogenic foci
Lymphoma	2nd, 3rd, 4th	Hypoechoic	Can vary	Irregular	Yes
Metastasis	Any	Hypoechoic		Irregular	Yes
Lipoma	3rd	Hyperechoic homogenous	Can vary	Sharp	No
Brunner gland hyperplasia	2nd or 3rd	Iso/Hyperechoic homogenous (less then lipoma)		Sharp	No

Table 2.
Main ultrasonographic characteristics of duodenal lesions.

standard [10]. As literature regarding duodenal SETs is scarce, there is no consensus about when to perform EUS-FNA, but as previously mentioned, EUS can perform poorly in diagnosing small lesions, so biopsies should be performed in all lesions that are considered suspicious (possible malignant or with malignity potential). All lesions of the fourth layer (muscularis propria) should be biopsied, as most gastrointestinal mesenchymal tumors (GIMTs) have these characteristics. Techniques to obtain deep biopsies, like "jumbo" or "buttonhole" biopsies, may have better outcomes than EUS-FNA in submucosal lesions, but carry high risk of hemorrhage [9, 11].

3. Lesions of the duodenal wall

3.1 Vascular lesions

Anechoic SETs account for a large number of different possible diagnoses. Doppler-color ultrasonography is the best method to differentiate between vascular and cystic lesions. Vascular lesions in the duodenum are most frequently varices;

other vascular malformations are rare. Varices are located in the third layer (submucosa) and are anechoic. Even in the absence of Doppler facilities, varices can be diagnosed by following their course, identifying other collateral vessels and perforating veins. Small varices can be compressed by the tip of the echoendoscope and misdiagnosed, so it is important to be careful. Therapeutic interventions like cyanoacrylate injection or coiling can be EUS guided.

3.2 Cystic and mixed lesions

Cystic tumors are liquid-filled cavities, hence anechogenic, that present in many different shapes and sizes. Many different lesions can present themselves as cystic or cystic-like. The most used classifications are simple cystic, polycystic or mixed (with liquid and solid components) [8].

3.2.1 Duplication cysts

Cysts are rounded, unilocular and clearly delineated, with a completely anechoic content and dorsal enhancement. The most common diagnosis is a duplication cyst, which forms from a maldevelopment of the gut. Duplication cysts are located in the third layer (submucosa) and have a characteristic duplication of all the layers of the gut wall. They have a low risk of malignant transformation, or they can become symptomatic following increasing in size, infection or rupture. EUS-FNA is rarely needed when the diagnosis is unclear.

3.2.2 Brunner's gland hyperplasia

Brunner's glands are found in the duodenum and have an alkaline secretion, neutralizing stomach acid. Hyperplasia of these glands is usually asymptomatic, but can give a polyposis-like duodenum. The cause is thought to be excessive stimulation from excessive gastric acids, chronic inflammation or the decrease of pancreatic function. They are located mainly, if not exclusively, in the duodenal bulb [5].

Echoendoscopic appearance can vary as isoechoic or hyperechoic, sometimes with cysts inside. They arise from the third layer (submucosa) and much more rarely from the second one (deep mucosa). The diagnosis is based on biopsy result (**Figure 1**).

3.2.3 Lymphangiomas

Lymphangiomas consist of multiple dilated lymphatic vessels situated mostly in the third layer (submucosa), rarely in the second layer (mucosa). They are thought to be benign malformations of the lymphatic system that form a mass in the digestive tract. Lymphangiectasias, in contrast, are dilations of existing mucosal lymphatic vessels and described endoscopically as multiple small, white polyp-like elevations in the duodenum. They are mainly found in the small intestine, have a polyp-like appearance and are soft and easily compressible with a normal overlying mucosa. Most are asymptomatic; rarely, the size can cause obstruction, abdominal pain and hemorrhage [12]. As previously mentioned, they are formed from dilated lymphatic vessels, but also from smooth muscle fibers and connective tissue. Endosonographically they most often appear as polycystic. Their appearance varies vastly depending on the amount of smooth muscle and connective tissue. When they take up a large share of the lymphangioma it appears inhomogeneous, rather than anechoic.

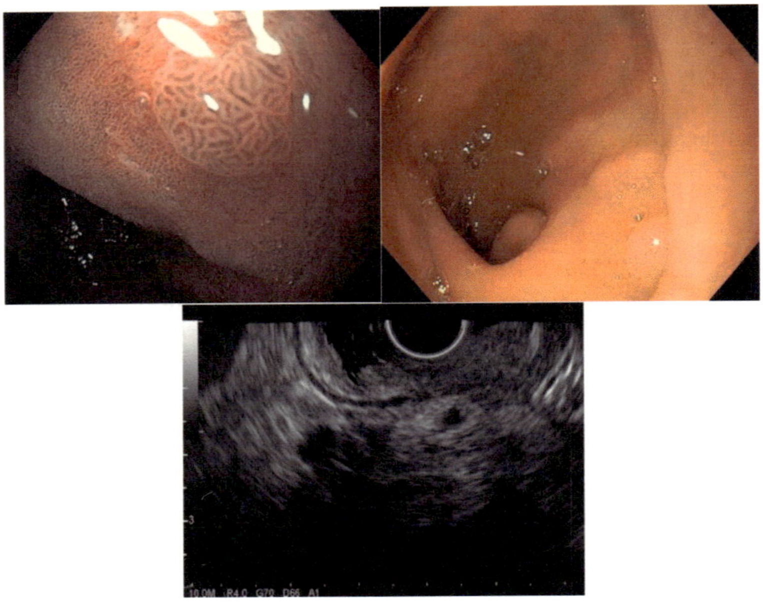

Figure 1.
Endoscopic (top row) and ultrasonographic (bottom row) appearance of Brunner's gland hyperplasia.

3.2.4 Pancreatic rest

Pancreatic rest, also known as heterotopic pancreatic tissue or ectopic pancreas, is pancreatic tissue located, aberrantly, in the digestive tract wall, most often in the stomach. It is usually asymptomatic and is an incidental finding at EGD or CT scan. Its endoscopic characteristics are irregular overlaying mucosa and a central umbilication. Rests originate from the third and fourth layer (submucosa and muscularis propria) and their sonographic appearance is most often mixed (solid and liquid) but highly variable, depending on the dominant tissue. Type 1 heterotopia consists of both pancreatic acini and ducts. Type 2 consists solely of pancreatic acini, and type 3 of pancreatic ducts. Types 1 and 2 have a hypoechoic, inhomogeneous sonographic appearance, poorly delineated from the surrounding tissue (secondary to the lobulated structure of acinous tissue). Type 3 most often appears as a septated cyst (multiple dilated pancreatic ducts). A characteristic appearance of a pancreatic rest seems to be thickening of the fourth layer behind the mass (muscularis propria) [13]. Asymptomatic lesions should be followed endoscopically for size changes, and the rare cases of symptomatic lesions can be resected endoscopically by snare, band ligation or more advanced resection techniques. If the muscularis propria is involved and the heterotopic tissue must be removed, surgical resection is preferred [14].

3.3 Solid lesions

3.3.1 Lipomas

Lipomas are the most frequent solid, hyperechoic SETs in the duodenum. They are composed of mature lipocytes and originate from the third layer (the submucosa). They are most common in the colon, but are also in the stomach and small bowel. A characteristic endoscopic appearance, with a yellowish tint and a typical indent when compressing it with a biopsy forceps ("pillow" sign), does not need follow-up with EUS.

Echoendoscopically lipomas are hyperechoic, homogenous, arise from the third layer and are very well differentiated from the other layers with a clear margin. This typical appearance does not need histological evaluation (EUS-FNA).

Lipomas do not need treatment/resection or follow-up when they have a typical appearance and are asymptomatic (**Figure 2**).

3.3.2 GISTs

GISTs are the most common mesenchymal tumors in the GI tract, most often found in the stomach and much more rarely in the duodenum. They originate from the pacemaker cells of the digestive tract wall, the interstitial cells of Cajal. They are a class of SETs that present the most difficulties in diagnosis and management: hypoechoic SETs that originate from the muscle layers (mainly the muscularis propria, sometimes muscularis mucosae). They are similar in sonographic structure and mesenchymal origin. The molecular particularity of GISTs is a mutation in the gene that codes the c-Kit protein. More than 95% of them are immunohistochemical CD117 positive [15]. All GISTs have malignant potential, with the main factors influencing prognosis being mitotic rate, size and location (small intestinal GISTs seem to have a worse prognosis than gastric ones). The most common first symptom is GI bleeding, but a large number of GISTs are probably asymptomatic, as they are a common finding in postmortem examinations or in gastric resection specimens. GISTs in the small intestine may be more aggressive than those located in the stomach, (40–50% of GISTs in the small intestine are malignant, compared with 20–25% of gastric GISTs) [16].

Endoscopically their appearance is similar to other SETs; a bulge in the wall of the digestive tract with normal overlaying mucosa. Sometimes there is a central ulceration or inflammation of the mucosa. They are hypoechoic, arising from a muscle layer. The large ones most often arise from the fourth layer (the muscularis propria). Leiomyomas and other mesenchymal tumors, like the schwannoma, have a similar appearance, but are benign. Therefore a correct diagnosis is essential before a therapeutic decision. Location can be the best indicator of a hypoechoic SET. In the duodenum they mostly turn out to be neuroendocrine tumors. More rarely they are GISTs or granular cell tumors, and they are almost never leiomyomas.

All GISTs have malignant potential, so even though small GISTs used to be followed endoscopically, the current trend is to remove all GISTs. Differentiating between a GIST and a leiomyoma is difficult, even with EUS-FNA/FNB sometimes, thus contrast enhancement is helpful in such cases.

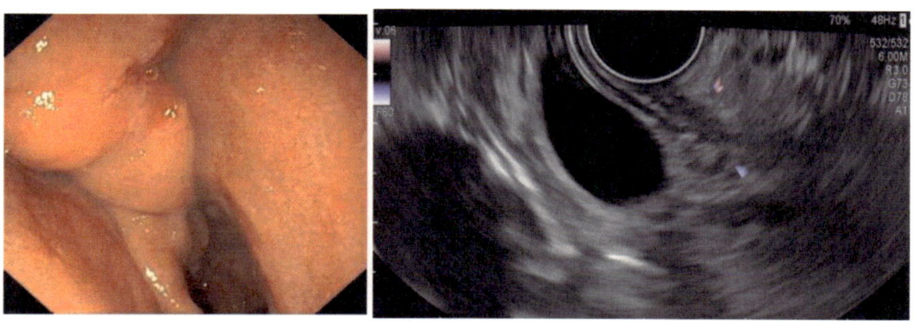

Figure 2.
Endoscopic (left) and ultrasonographic (right) appearance of a duodenal lipoma.

There is no specific study on contrast enhancement in case of duodenal SETs. A meta-analysis of gastric and esophageal SETs showed that contrast-enhanced endoscopic ultrasound is able to discriminate between GISTs and benign SETs with a pooled sensitivity of 89% and a specificity of 82%. For differentiating the malignant potential of GISTs, the sensitivity was 96% and the specificity was 53% [17]. An uptake of the contrast with the vascular hilum present suggests a leiomyoma, but a heterogenous vascularity suggests GISTs while irregular vessels suggest malignant GISTs.

3.3.3 Neuroendocrine tumors (NETs)

NETs (also known as carcinoid tumors) are mostly asymptomatic tumors with endocrine cell origin. Mostly, they are discovered incidentally, but they can cause hemorrhage, abdominal pain or syndromes related to functional active substances

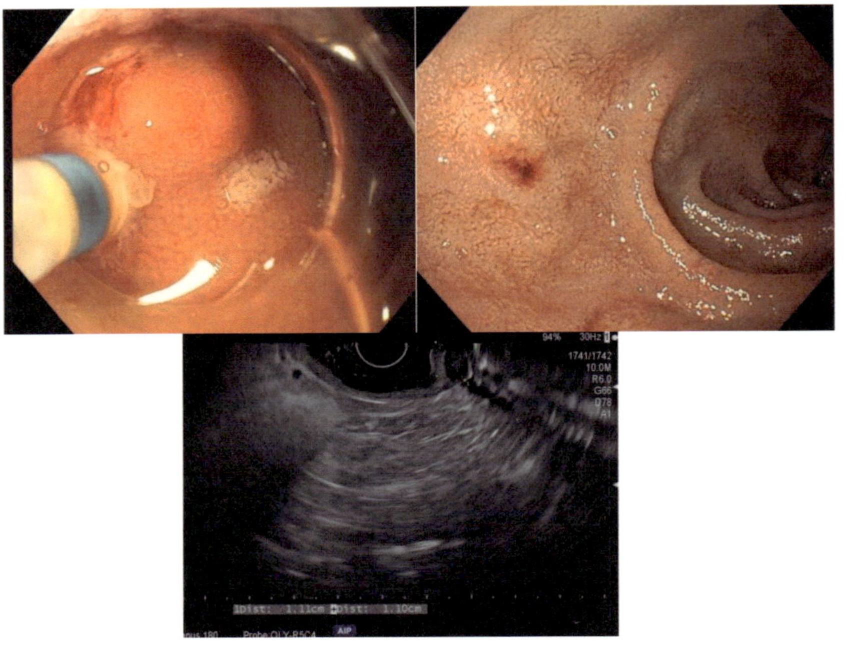

Figure 3.
(A) Endoscopic appearance during cap-assisted resection of a duodenal NET. (B) Same lesion after resection. (C) Echoendoscopic appearance of the same duodenal NET (hypoechoic, well delineated).

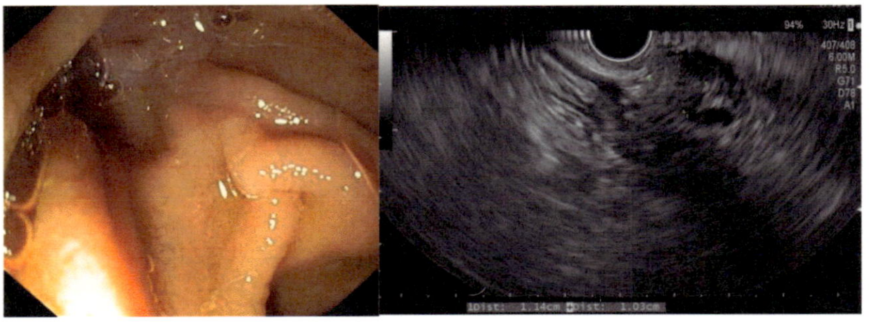

Figure 4.
Endoscopic (left) and ultrasonographic (right) appearance of the papilla.

secreted by them. They are found along the GI tract, more often in the rectum or stomach, but also in the small intestine.

Their endoscopic appearance is not characteristic, usually resembling a small polypoid lesion with normal overlaying mucosa. Endosonographically they are mostly hypoechoic or isoechoic, and arise from the second layer (mucosa), but can extend to the third layer (submucosa).

The variety of histological types, sizes and location origins, combined with the risk of malignant transformation, illustrate the necessity to resect NETs. In principle, if the lesion is smaller than 1 cm and does not invade the muscularis propria, endoscopic resection is possible, otherwise surgical resection is recommended (**Figure 3**).

3.3.4 Major and minor papilla lesions

The upstream ducts are well recognized. Following the duodenal wall, especially the muscularis major papilla represents the opening into the duodenum of the common bile duct and pancreatic duct. The tumor of the papilla is very well visualized during EUS and the dilatation of the propria can differentiate small ampullary tumors that are limited to papilla from distal common bile duct tumors, which are situated beyond the muscularis propria layer (**Figure 4**).

The pancreatic accessory duct arrives in the duodenum at the level of the minor papilla. Sometimes EGD can confound it with an SET [4]. EUS examination can easily differentiate it from a tumor, as it is not part of the duodenal wall and the secondary duct is visible arriving at this level.

3.3.5 Adenomas

Adenomas can appear in the duodenum, as anywhere else in the GI tract, sporadically or part of polyposis syndromes. They are premalignant lesions that usually necessitate removal. Peri-papillary location makes resection techniques more problematic, as simple resection can cause damage to the pancreatic or biliary ducts. Because they are mucosal lesions (second layer), solely EGD can be used for management. However, EUS can be necessary in certain circumstances, such as evaluating the depth of invasion if a malignancy is suspected, guiding the choice of treatment method (lesions extending to the submucosa need more advanced endoscopic resection techniques or surgery) and evaluating intraductal extension in peri-papillary lesions (**Figure 5**).

3.3.6 Malignant tumors

Malignant tumors of the duodenal wall are rare. Possible malignant tumors identified at this level include adenocarcinomas (from adenomas), malignant mesenchymal tumors (malignant GISTs), malignant NETs, lymphomas and metastases from other cancers (very rare).

These tumors share a common endosonographic characteristic by not respecting the layers of the duodenal wall (which are often lost) and often have adjacent lymphadenopathies.

3.4 Uncommon duodenal SETs

3.4.1 Leiomyomas

Leiomyomas are truly benign tumors arising from smooth muscle tissue, that is, the fourth layer and more rarely the second (muscularis mucosae). They are

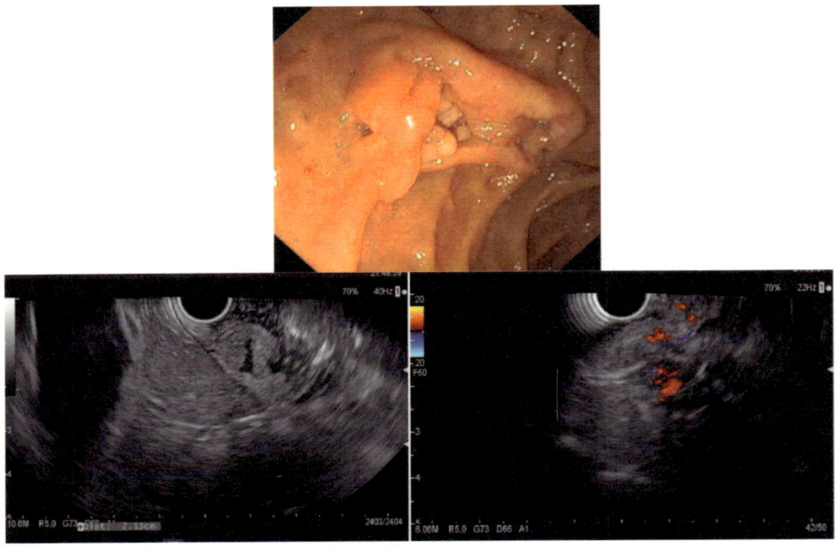

Figure 5.
Top: Endoscopic view of duodenal adenoma. Bottom: Echoendoscopic appearance of the same adenomas. Enhanced vascularization is visible.

mostly found in the esophagus, but they are described all over the GI tract. Their hypoechoic sonographic appearance makes them difficult to distinguish from other GIMTs. As such, EUS-FNA and histological examination are needed for a correct diagnosis. Resection is necessary only in case of symptoms.

3.4.2 Granular cell tumors

Granular cell tumors (also known as schwannomas) are benign lesions that arise from the peripheral nerve sheath. They are hypoechoic, homogenous, well delineated and arise from the second or third layer of the duodenum (submucosa or muscularis propria). Even though the endosonographic appearance makes them hard to differentiate from GISTs or leiomyomas, schwannomas are much more rarely encountered in the GI tract. Tissue acquisition discriminates the diagnosis in such situations.

3.4.3 Fibroid polyps

Fibroid polyps are rare inflammatory tumors, sometimes found in the duodenum. They arise from the second or third layers and are usually hyperechoic and inhomogeneous [18].

3.4.4 Hematomas

Duodenal hematomas have been described, especially after abdominal trauma. However, some are spontaneous or arise from complications of endoscopic biopsies or other invasive maneuvers. They are usually diagnosed by CT scan or EGD. EUS is only needed in cases when the diagnosis is unclear, which is rare. They arise from the deep layers of the mucosa or submucosa (second or third layer). They have a different sonographic appearance depending on when they are evaluated. Initially, they have a heterogenous appearance in the first 24 hrs, which turns hyperechoic as more clots are formed and then slowly turns hypoechoic over the following weeks as it resorbs.

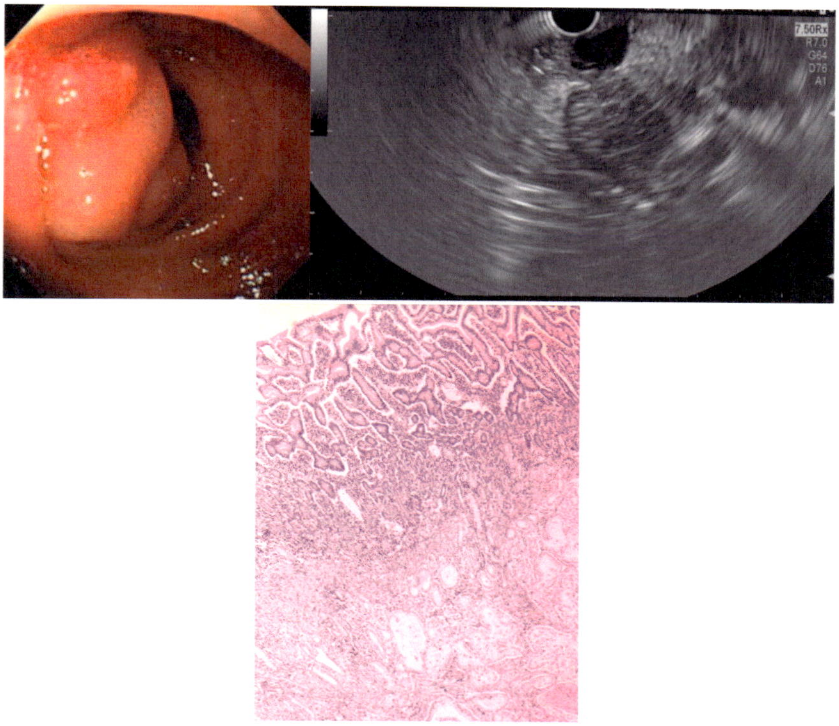

Figure 6.
(A) Endoscopic view of external compression in the duodenum. (B) The echoendoscopic view shows an anechogenic lesion close to the transducer, a cyst. The pancreatic parenchima shows modifications consistent with chronic pancreatitis. (C) EUS-FNA - Paraduodenal cyst lined by inflammation and granulation tissue with no epitheliallining (HE-5X).

3.4.5 Gangliocytic paraganglioma

Gangliocytic paragangliomas are GI mesenchymal tumors, most often found in the second part of the duodenum near the ampulla of Vater [19]. They are formed by a varying mixture of spindle cells, epithelioid cells and ganglion cells (cells found also in other GIMTs). They are located in the third layer (submucosa) and are hypoechoic and homogenous. Histology usually offers the final diagnosis, as hypoechoic SETs are hard to distinguish on EUS alone.

3.5 Extrinsic compressions

In a series of 169 suspected SETs in the duodenum, which were referred to EUS, 12 were extrinsic compressions, with seven from the gallbladder and five from the pancreas [4]. EUS is very efficient in these cases, as it can identify the layers of the duodenum wall and correctly identify the duodenal compression as being extrinsic, as well as determine the cause of the compression and/or invasion (**Figures 6** and 7).

4. EUS tissue acquisition

The sampling of SELs is unnecessary in case of lipoma or duplication cyst. However, some duodenal SETs (GISTs, neuroendocrine tumors) have malignant potential, so the size of the lesion is not a limitation for tissue acquisition. The

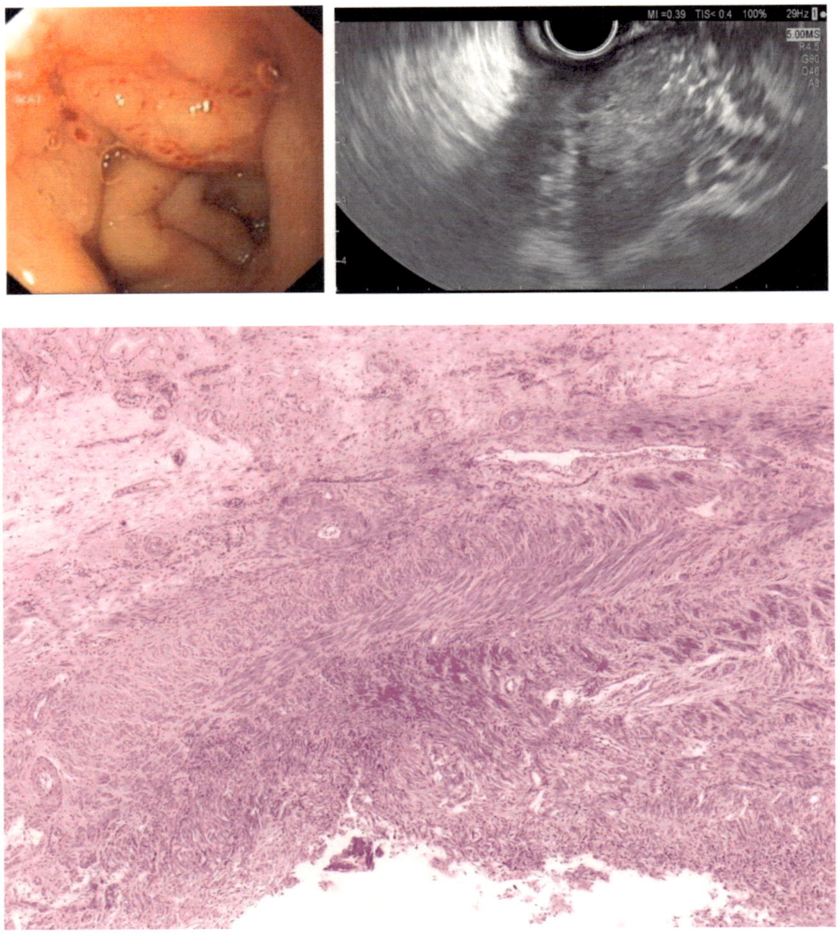

Figure 7.
External invasion from a pancreatic head adenocarcinoma. (A) Endoscopic view: There are mucosal modifications visible (as opposed to 6A). (B) Echoendoscopic view confirms there is a pancreatic tumor. (C) EUS-FNA - foci of pancreatic ductal adenocarcinoma infiltrating submucosa of the duodenal wall (HE-5X).

accuracy of EUS alone compared to the final histology (ESD or surgical specimen) varies between 44% and 66% and tissue acquisition is important for a correct diagnosis [20–22].

The sampling has to be performed using bite-to-bite biopsy followed by mucosal resection or submucosal resection in case of the lesions belonging to the second or third layers [11]. In case of the lesions originating from the fourth layer, the indication is for EUS-FNA or EUS–fine-needle biopsy (EUS-FNB) [23]. The unroofing method for sampling of fourth-layer lesions of gastric location was compared to EUS-FNB, but no difference for histologic core procurement was noted [24].

EUS sampling is preferred in case of lesions situated in the third or fourth layer, because the risk of bleeding is usually low and seeding into the peritoneum is avoided compared to percutaneous biopsy.

However, the use of EUS-FNA, especially with 22-guage and 25-guage needles, gave a diagnostic rate of 60% in a meta-analysis of 978 patients [25]. The main limitation is difficulty in assessing the architecture of the lesion sampled and the mitotic index. No influence of SET size on the diagnostic rate of FNA was found in a retrospective study of 112 patients [26]. The use of a pro-core needle compared to FNA needles does not improve the diagnostic rate [27–30]. However, only one study included SETs from the duodenum [29]. The use of FNB gave better accuracy than EUS-FNA (88.03% vs. 77.19% [P = .030]) or EUS-FNA plus rapid on-site evaluation (ROSE) (87.25% vs. 68.00% [P = .024]), but no difference was noted compared to EUS-FNB plus ROSE [31]. In a meta-analysis comprising 10 studies that compared EUS-FNB and EUS-FNA, the diagnostic accuracy was greater in patients undergoing FNB sampling (OR, 4.10; 95% CI, 2.48–6.79; P < .0001) with a fewer number of passes and higher rate of optimal core procurement (OR, 3.27; 95% CI, 2.03–5.27; P < .0001) [32]. Because the distal duodenum can be difficult to reach, the sampling from this location is feasible with thinner 25G needles, with a definitive diagnosis in 88% of patients.

5. Conclusions

EUS is essential for evaluating duodenal lesions correctly and completely. EUS can identify if the lesion originates from the mucosa or the deeper layers of the duodenal wall, or if it is extrinsic. Other diagnostic methods lack the resolution to distinguish between them correctly. In addition, EUS can obtain tissue for histological analysis in all cases, as EGD-guided biopsies are not deep enough for SETs. Choice of treatment is also decided following EUS, as benign lesions do not need removal, potential malignant lesions (NETs, GISTs) can be followed or resected and malignant lesions can be resected endoscopically if EUS does not identify invasion of the deeper layers. Given all this, along with the complex surroundings of the duodenum, its thin walls and the difficult anatomical position for surgical interventions, EUS is crucial in lesions of the duodenal wall.

Conflict of interest

The authors declare no conflict of interest.

Author details

Andrada Seicean[1]*, Voicu Rednic[2] and Radu Seicean[3]

1 University of Medicine and Pharmacy "Iuliu Hațieganu," Regional Institute of Gastroenterology "Prof. Dr. Octavian Fodor," Cluj-Napoca, Romania

2 Regional Institute of Gastroenterology "Prof. Dr. Octavian Fodor," Cluj-Napoca, Romania

3 University of Medicine and Pharmacy "Iuliu Hațieganu," County Emergency Hospital, Cluj-Napoca, Romania

*Address all correspondence to: andradaseicean@gmail.com

IntechOpen

© 2021 The Author(s). Licensee IntechOpen. This chapter is distributed under the terms of the Creative Commons Attribution License (http://creativecommons.org/licenses/by/3.0), which permits unrestricted use, distribution, and reproduction in any medium, provided the original work is properly cited.

References

[1] Hizawa K, Kawasaki M, Kouzuki T, Suekane H, Matsumoto T, Fujishima M. Endosonographic classications of gastrointestinal submucosal tumors. Dig Endosc [Internet]. 2000 Apr 1;12(2):120-5. Available from: https://doi.org/10.1046/j.1443-1661.2000.00020.x

[2] Jenssen C, Dietrich CF. Endoscopic ultrasound of gastrointestinal subepithelial lesions. Ultraschall Med [Internet]. 2008 Jun;29(3):236-256; quiz 257—64. Available from: https://doi.org/10.1055/s-2008-1027388

[3] Chen TK, Wu CH, Lee CL, Lai YC, Yang SS, Tu TC. Endoscopic ultrasonography to study the causes of extragastric compression mimicking gastric submucosal tumor. J Formos Med Assoc. 2001 Nov;100(11):758-761.

[4] Xu G, Wu Y, Wang L, Chen H. Values of endoscopic ultrasonography for diagnosis and treatment of duodenal protruding lesions. J Zhejiang Univ Sci B. 2008 Apr;9(4):329-334.

[5] Pavlovic Markovic A, Rösch T, Alempijevic T, Krstic M, Tomic D, Dugalic P, et al. Endoscopic ultrasound for differential diagnosis of duodenal lesions. Ultraschall Med. 2012 Dec;33(7):E210–E217.

[6] Kawamoto K, Yamada Y, Utsunomiya T, Okamura H, Mizuguchi M, Motooka M, et al. Gastrointestinal submucosal tumors: evaluation with endoscopic US. Radiology. 1997 Dec;205(3):733-740.

[7] Sonnenberg A, Amorosi SL, Lacey MJ, Lieberman DA. Patterns of endoscopy in the United States: analysis of data from the Centers for Medicare and Medicaid Services and the National Endoscopic Database. Gastrointest Endosc. 2008 Mar;67(3):489-496.

[8] Dietrich CF. Endoscopic Ultrasound: An Introductory Manual and Atlas. 2nd ed. Thieme; 2011. 1280 p.

[9] Cantor MJ, Davila RE, Faigel DO. Yield of tissue sampling for subepithelial lesions evaluated by EUS: a comparison between forceps biopsies and endoscopic submucosal resection. Gastrointest Endosc. 2006 Jul;64(1):29-34.

[10] Karaca C, Turner BG, Cizginer S, Forcione D, Brugge W. Accuracy of EUS in the evaluation of small gastric subepithelial lesions. Gastrointest Endosc. 2010 Apr;71(4):722-727.

[11] Buscaglia JM, Nagula S, Jayaraman V, Robbins DH, Vadada D, Gross SA, et al. Diagnostic yield and safety of jumbo biopsy forceps in patients with subepithelial lesions of the upper and lower GI tract. Gastrointest Endosc. 2012 Jun;75(6):1147-1152.

[12] Rai P, Rao RN, Chakraborthy SBD. Caecal lymphangioma: a rare cause of gastrointestinal blood loss. BMJ Case Rep [Internet]. 2013 Apr 19;2013:bcr2013008866. Available from: http://casereports.bmj.com/content/2013/bcr-2013-008866.abstract

[13] Matsushita M, Hajiro K, Okazaki K, Takakuwa H. Gastric aberrant pancreas: EUS analysis in comparison with the histology. Gastrointest Endosc. 1999 Apr;49(4 Pt 1):493-497.

[14] Faulx AL, Kothari S, Acosta RD, Agrawal D, Bruining DH, Chandrasekhara V, et al. The role of endoscopy in subepithelial lesions of the GI tract. Gastrointest Endosc [Internet]. 2017 Jun 1;85(6):1117-32. Available from: https://doi.org/10.1016/j.gie.2017.02.022

[15] Rodriguez SA, Faigel DO. Endoscopic diagnosis of gastrointestinal

stromal cell tumors. Curr Opin Gastroenterol. 2007 Sep;23(5):539-543.

[16] Miettinen M, Lasota J. Gastrointestinal stromal tumors: pathology and prognosis at different sites. Semin Diagn Pathol. 2006 May;23(2):70-83.

[17] Tang JY, Tao KG, Zhang LY, Wu KM, Shi J, Zeng X, et al. Value of contrast-enhanced harmonic endoscopic ultrasonography in differentiating between gastrointestinal stromal tumors: A meta-analysis. J Dig Dis. 2019 Mar;20(3):127-134.

[18] Matsushita M, Hajiro K, Okazaki K, Takakuwa H. Gastric inflammatory fibroid polyps: endoscopic ultrasonographic analysis in comparison with the histology. Gastrointest Endosc. 1997 Jul;46(1):53-57.

[19] Loew BJ, Lukens FJ, Navarro F, Roy M, Mattia A, Howell DA. Successful endoscopic resection of a gangliocytic paraganglioma of the minor papilla in a patient with pancreas divisum and pancreatitis (with video). Gastrointest Endosc. 2007 Mar;65(3):547-550.

[20] Hwang JH, Saunders MD, Rulyak SJ, Shaw S, Nietsch H, Kimmey MB. A prospective study comparing endoscopy and EUS in the evaluation of GI subepithelial masses. Gastrointest Endosc. 2005 Aug;62(2):202-208.

[21] Lim TW, Choi CW, Kang DH, Kim HW, Park SB, Kim SJ. Endoscopic ultrasound without tissue acquisition has poor accuracy for diagnosing gastric subepithelial tumors. Medicine (Baltimore). 2016 Nov;95(44):e5246.

[22] Kim SY, Shim K-N, Lee J-H, Lim JY, Kim TO, Choe AR, et al. Comparison of the Diagnostic Ability of Endoscopic Ultrasonography and Abdominopelvic Computed Tomography in the Diagnosis of Gastric Subepithelial Tumors. Clin Endosc [Internet]. 2019 Nov;52(6):565-573. Available from: https://europepmc.org/articles/PMC6900302

[23] Cho JW. Current Guidelines in the Management of Upper Gastrointestinal Subepithelial Tumors. Clin Endosc. 2016 May;49(3):235-240.

[24] Park J, Park JC, Jo JH, Kim EH, Shin SK, Lee SK, et al. Prospective comparative study of endoscopic ultrasonography-guided fine-needle biopsy and unroofing biopsy. Dig liver Dis Off J Ital Soc Gastroenterol Ital Assoc Study Liver. 2019 Jun;51(6):831-836.

[25] Zhang X-C, Li Q-L, Yu Y-F, Yao L-Q, Xu M-D, Zhang Y-Q, et al. Diagnostic efficacy of endoscopic ultrasound-guided needle sampling for upper gastrointestinal subepithelial lesions: a meta-analysis. Surg Endosc. 2016 Jun;30(6):2431-2441.

[26] Hoda KM, Rodriguez SA, Faigel DO. EUS-guided sampling of suspected GI stromal tumors. Gastrointest Endosc. 2009 Jun;69(7):1218-1223.

[27] Iwai T, Kida M, Imaizumi H, Miyazawa S, Okuwaki K, Yamauchi H, et al. Randomized crossover trial comparing EUS-guided fine-needle aspiration with EUS-guided fine-needle biopsy for gastric subepithelial tumors. Diagn Cytopathol. 2018 Mar;46(3):228-233.

[28] Han JP, Lee TH, Hong SJ, Kim HK, Noh HM, Lee YN, et al. EUS-guided FNA and FNB after on-site cytological evaluation in gastric subepithelial tumors. J Dig Dis. 2016 Sep;17(9):582-587.

[29] Kim DH, Kim GH, Cho CM, Park CH, Na S-Y, Kim TH, et al. Feasibility of a 20-gauge ProCore needle in EUS-guided subepithelial tumor sampling: a prospective multicenter study. BMC Gastroenterol. 2018 Oct;18(1):151.

[30] Lee JH, Cho CJ, Park YS, Ahn JY, Kim DH, Na HK, et al. EUS-guided 22-gauge fine needle biopsy for the diagnosis of gastric subepithelial tumors larger than 2 cm. Scand J Gastroenterol [Internet]. 2016;51(4):486-493. Available from: https://doi.org/10.3109/00365521.2015.1052095

[31] de Moura DTH, McCarty TR, Jirapinyo P, Ribeiro IB, Flumignan VK, Najdawai F, et al. EUS-guided fine-needle biopsy sampling versus FNA in the diagnosis of subepithelial lesions: a large multicenter study. Gastrointest Endosc [Internet]. 2020 Jul;92(1):108-119.e3. Available from: https://doi.org/10.1016/j.gie.2020.02.021

[32] Facciorusso A, Sunny SP, Del Prete V, Antonino M, Muscatiello N. Comparison between fine-needle biopsy and fine-needle aspiration for EUS-guided sampling of subepithelial lesions: a meta-analysis. Gastrointest Endosc. 2020 Jan;91(1):14-22.e2.

Section 5

Intra-operative Endoscopy

Chapter 6

Role of Intraoperative Endoscopy in the Management of Small Bowel Diseases

Rahul Gupta, Arvind K. Singh, Jyoti Gupta and Houssem Ammar

Abstract

With the advances in the endoscopic technology, most of the small bowel diseases are being diagnosed by capsule endoscopy and device assisted enteroscopy. However, there are many clinical situations such as small bowel obstruction, foreign body impaction were these advanced endoscopic procedures cannot be performed. In such cases, intraoperative endoscopy plays a vital role in the management of these small bowel diseases. Intraoperative endoscopy is also very useful in identification of the site of obscure gastrointestinal bleeding in difficult cases. Moreover, capsule endoscopy and device assisted enteroscopy are expensive procedures and not readily available at all medical centers especially in low income countries. On the other hand, intraoperative endoscopy can be easily performed by conventional gastroscope and colonoscope. In this chapter, we have discussed the indications, techniques, outcomes and complications of intraoperative endoscopy in the current era of deep enteroscopy.

Keywords: intraoperative endoscopy, enteroscopy, inflammatory bowel disease, Peutz-Jeghers syndrome, Crohn's disease

1. Introduction

Traditionally, intraoperative endoscopy (IOE) was the only means for the visualization of small bowel mucosal lesions not accessible to upper gastrointestinal endoscopy and colonoscopy. However, with the advances in abdominal imaging and the advent of capsule endoscopy (CE), the use of IOE diminished. A comparative study of CE and IOE found the sensitivity and specificity of CE to be 95% and 75%, respectively [1]. Hence, most guidelines recommend CE for detection of suspected small bowel lesions in patients with obscure gastrointestinal (GI) bleed. However, the main disadvantage of CE was inability to perform therapeutic procedures. Subsequently, the device assisted enteroscopy (DAE), namely, spiral endoscopy, double balloon enteroscopy (DBE) and single balloon enteroscopy (SBE) was developed which has brought paradigm shift in the treatment of small bowel mucosal diseases. DAE allows visualization, biopsy and removal of the small bowel mucosal lesions.

However, IOE is still an indispensable tool for the evaluation and treatment of small bowel diseases in special situations and institutions with lack of DAE

IntechOpen

Advantages of IOE	Disadvantages of IOE
Complete bowel examination is possible in same sitting	Anesthesia and laparotomy related complications
The procedure is safe as it is performed under direct vision	Enterotomy related complications
Allows peritoneal, mesentery and omental examination and biopsy, if required	Availability of the endoscopy equipments and endoscopist at the time of surgery
Allows definitive treatment of the disease in the same sitting	Inability to negotiate the endoscope in case of dense bowel adhesions
Minimizes the number of procedures and enterotomies in patients with multiple lesions like PJS	Inability to visualize the mucosa in case of massive bleeding

Table 1.
Advantages and disadvantages of intraoperative endoscopy.

facilities. The reported success rate of IOE to achieve complete enteroscopy ranges between 57–100% in different series [1–10]. The advantages and disadvantages of IOE have been summarized in **Table 1**.

2. Indications

In the current era, despite the widespread use of DAE, IOE plays an important in the management of various GI disorders. In a 10-year study by Kopacova et al., the authors performed IOE in 41 patients with the commonest indication being obscure gastrointestinal bleeding followed by Peutz-Jeghers syndrome (PJS) [6]. The indications of IOE in the present scenario are as follows:

- Obscure gastrointestinal bleeding – It is recurrent or persistent bleeding from the unknown source in the GI tract that could not be identified on conventional endoscopy, colonoscopy and barium studies or enteroclysis [11]. Small bowel lesions account for 45–75% cases of obscure gastrointestinal bleed [11, 12]. In such cases, extensive investigations including enterography using computed tomography (CT) or magnetic resonance imaging (MRI), CE, DBE and RBC scan can often help in identifying the lesion (**Figure 1**). However, sometimes it is not possible to identify the site and cause of GI bleed in such patients despite exhaustive work-up. IOE is very helpful in detecting the mucosal lesions within the small bowel of patients with GI bleed (**Figure 2**). In a recent series of 67 patients with GI bleed, CE, colonoscopy, upper gastrointestinal endoscopy and DBE was performed in 96%, 87%, 87% and 73% cases respectively [10]. Despite these preoperative investigations, IOE was performed in 40% patients with the diagnostic yield of 76% [10].

- PJS – It is characterized by presence of multiple hamartomatous polyps throughout the GI tract, mucocutaneous pigmentation and an increased risk of GI cancers. These polyps are predominantly located in the small and can lead to several problems including recurrent abdominal pain, GI bleed, intussusception, bowel obstruction and perforation. As per the recommended guidelines, polyps more than 1 cm should be excised to prevent future complications [13]. Previously, these patients required surgical excision with or without IOE. But with the availability of DAE, many of these polyps can be removed endoscopically (**Figure 3**). Nevertheless, surgery and IOE is required

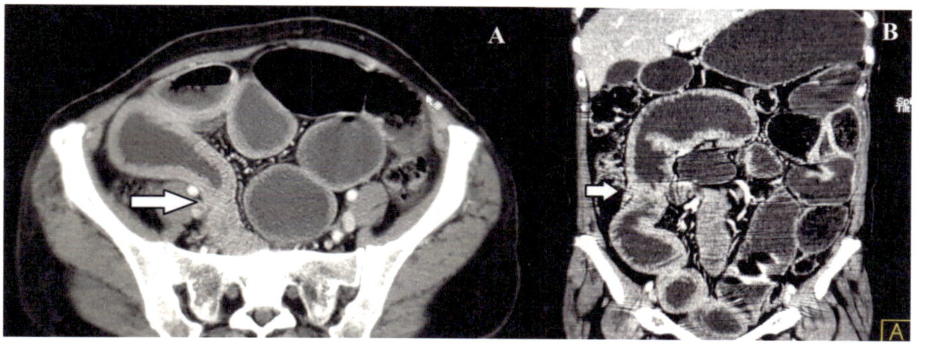

Figure 1.
Computed tomography - a 53-year-old lady presented with anemia, weight loss and recurrent abdominal pain for one year. On computed tomography, she was found to have thickening in the mid segment of the ileum (arrow) with proximal dilated bowel loops containing feculent material (A: Axial section, B – Coronal section).

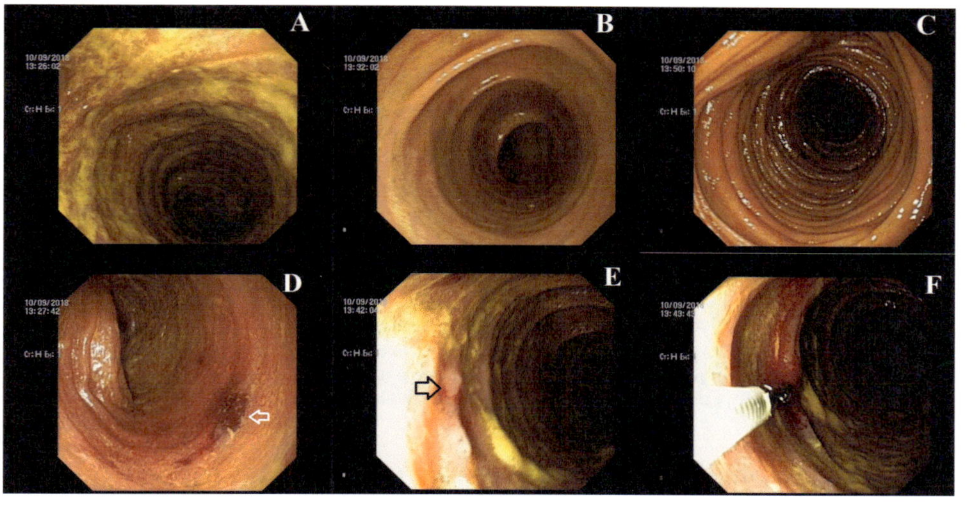

Figure 2.
Intraoperative enteroscopy via enterotomy of the patient with ileal thickening on computed tomography showing normal mucosal folds (A, B, C), a suspected vascular lesion (arrow, D), a small mucosal lesion (arrow, E) which was biopsied (F). No ileal stricture or significant mucosal disease was identified.

in many cases for complete exploration of small bowel and resection of large or malignant polyps (**Figure 4**). In a recent study of 27 patients with PJS, the success rate of enteroscopy was 76% [14]. IOE was required in 4 patients which improved the complete treatment rate to 92%. IOE has also been shown to facilitate polyp resection, reduce the number of laparotomies [6] and extensive bowel resection [15].

- Familial adenomatous polyposis (FAP) – It is an autosomal dominant disorder characterized by development of premalignant adenomatous polyps in the colon. Moreover, these patients are at the risk of development of duodenal polyposis, duodenal cancer, jejunal and ileal polyps [16]. Most of these can be visualized using conventional upper gastrointestinal endoscopy and colonoscopy. CE and DAE are useful for the visualization of jejunal and ileal polyps. However, in FAP patients with history of abdominal surgery such as pancreatoduodenectomy for duodenal cancer or total proctocolectomy for colorectal

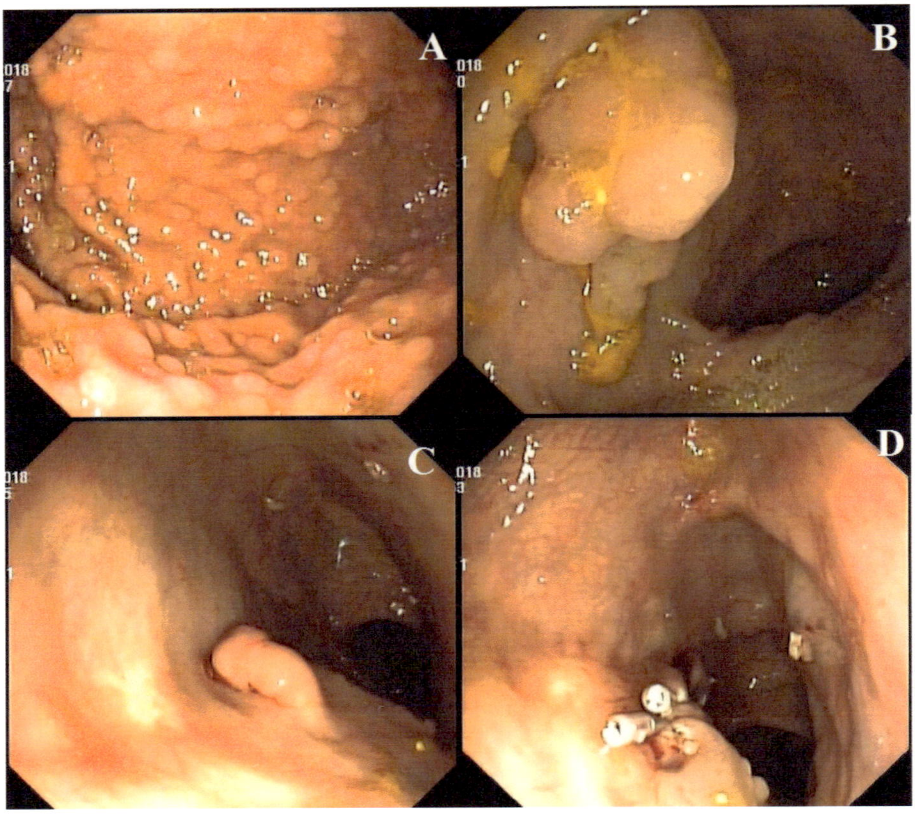

Figure 3.
Peutz-Jeghers syndrome – The follow-up gastroscopy of the patient with Peutz-Jeghers syndrome one year after intraoperative enteroscopy and polyp excision showing multiple small polyps throughout the stomach (A). Few pedunculated polyps were present in the large bowel (B, C) which were excised endoscopically (D).

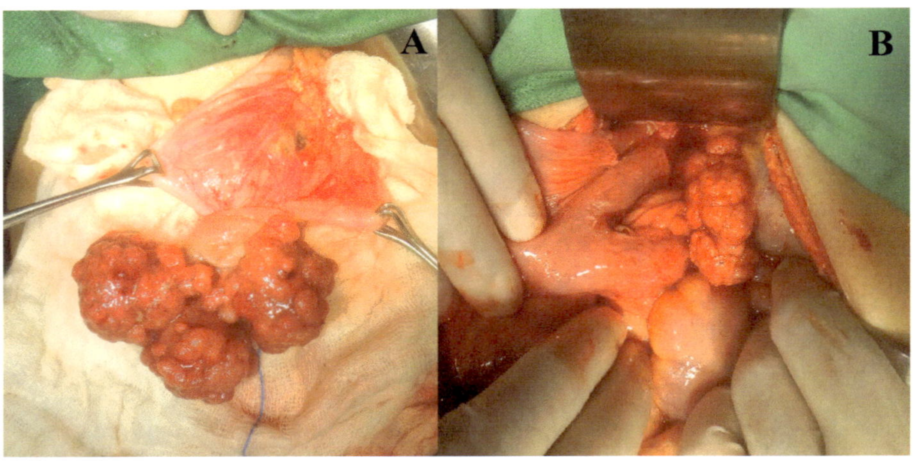

Figure 4.
Peutz-Jeghers syndrome – A 29-year-man presented with recurrent abdominal pain. On evaluation, he was found to have multiple polyps throughout the small and large intestine causing intussusception. At surgery, intraoperative enteroscopy via oral and anal route was performed and small polyps amenable to endoscopic resection were excised. Two large polyps, one in the transverse colon (A) and another in the proximal jejunum (B) were marked by endoscopy and excised surgically.

cancer, diagnostic and/or therapeutic DAE can be difficult. In such cases, IOE can be used to achieve complete clearance [16].

- Crohn's disease (CD) – It is an inflammatory bowel disease predominantly affecting the small intestine. The transmural inflammation leads to the development of deep ulcers causing GI bleeding and small bowel strictures causing intestinal obstruction. In presence of strictures, CE is contraindicated due to the risk of impaction. DAE also has its limitation in passing across the tight strictures making complete small bowel examination difficult. IOE helps in examining the mucosal side of the involved bowel segments to determine the disease activity. Previous studies involving CD patients have reported that IOE can identify new lesions not seen on preoperative examination [17].

Patients not responding to medical therapy or those who develop persistent GI bleeding or intestinal obstruction require surgical intervention. At surgery, multiple segments of small bowel with skip areas are often involved. The extent and type of surgery in such cases is difficult to ascertain. IOE allows complete small bowel examination and helps in surgical planning. In such cases, surgical intervention is most often performed for tight strictures (<15 mm diameter), stricture with active ulcer and bleeding ulcer [18].

IOE is also useful in CD patients undergoing emergency surgery for intestinal obstruction or perforation without prior endoscopic examination. In such cases, complete small bowel evaluation along with ileocecal junction is important to prevent postoperative complications and avoid repeated surgeries.

- Bowel obstruction or perforation – Sometimes, patients presenting with small bowel obstruction or perforation without prior endoscopic evaluation may require IOE for appropriate surgical treatment. One such situation is the presence of multiple strictures on preoperative CT. Similar to CD, patients with multiple strictures due to other causes such as tuberculosis requiring emergency surgery for intestinal obstruction or perforation can undergo IOE in the same sitting if feasible to allow complete small bowel examination and avoid multiple surgeries (**Figure 5**). Another clinical situation is difficulty in identification of the cause of bowel obstruction. In one of our previously reported cases, a patient of moderately severe acute gallstone pancreatitis developed colonic obstruction in the follow up [19]. On CT abdomen, there was a resolving peripancreatic collection surrounding the transverse colon with grossly dilated ascending colon and small bowel loops. In order to rule out mucosal disease, IOE via enterotomy route was performed (**Figure 6**). As there was no mucosal disease, side-to-side ileo-transverse colonic anastomosis was performed without colonic resection [19].

- Foreign body (FB) removal – Most of the cases of non-impacted FB ingestion can be managed conservatively. Sharp FB ingestion require endoscopic removal if feasible. Few cases with impacted FB in the small bowel not accessible to endoscopic removal or those who develop complications such as intestinal perforation require surgery.

Some cases with multiple FB ingestion located at different locations may require IOE to remove all the foreign bodies with minimum enterotomies. IOE can also help in such cases to confirm complete clearance during the operation [20].

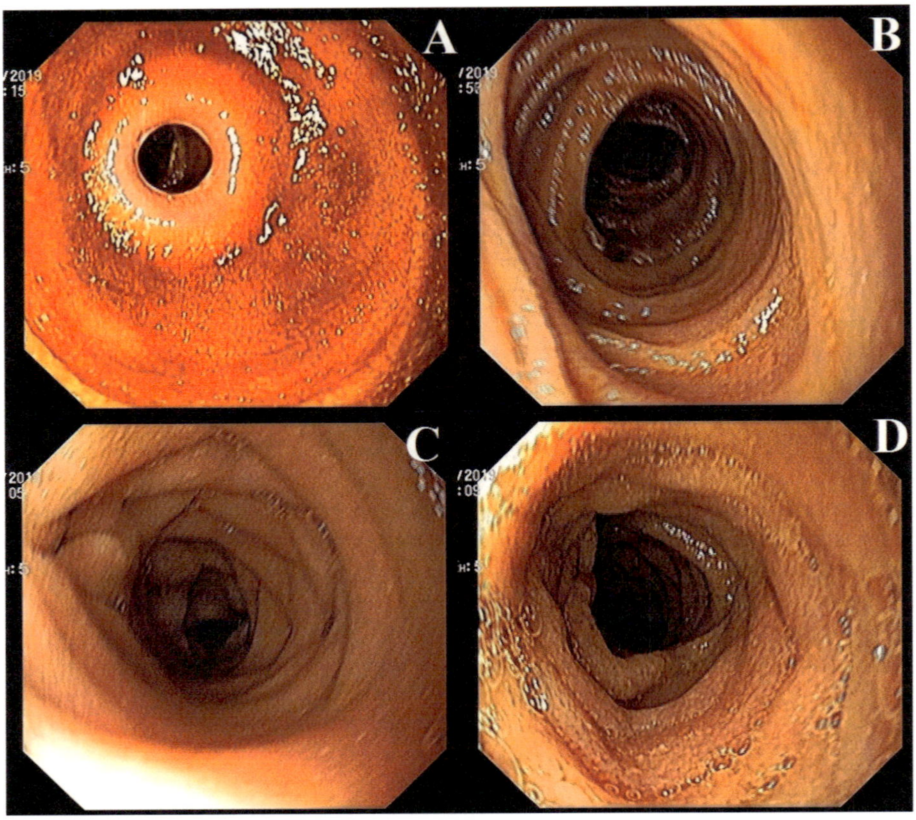

Figure 5.
Intraoperative enteroscopy via enterotomy of a patient with multiple small bowel strictures on computed tomography showing a narrow stricture in the proximal ileum (A). Rest of the small bowel showed mild mucosal edema at few places with no obvious strictures (B, C, D).

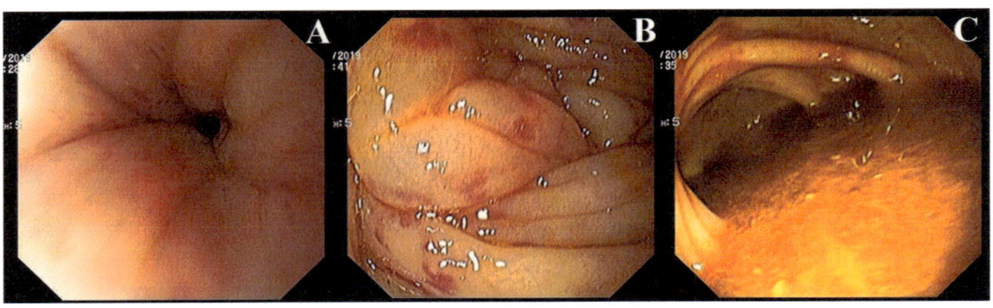

Figure 6.
Intraoperative enteroscopy via enterotomy of a patient with resolving acute pancreatitis and colonic obstruction showing mucosal edema at the site of obstruction (A, B) with grossly dilated colon loaded with feculent material (C).

- Failure of DAE to identify or treat the lesion – Often, complete small bowel examination is not possible with DAE. The reasons for failure of DAE include previous laparotomies, bowel adhesions, anatomical variations, etc. [21]. In such cases, IOE is useful in achieving complete bowel evaluation and treatment if required in the same sitting.

- Abdominal surgery required for other reasons – In some situations such as CD with symptomatic gallstone disease or FAP with periampullary carcinoma, if the patient is planned for abdominal surgery, then IOE can be performed in the same sitting instead of DAE.

- Identification of the site of disease during surgery – In the era of DAE, most of the small bowel lesions requiring surgical excision are marked with India ink. However, in some cases were the ink is not visible or cases were the mucosal lesions were detected on CE such as ectopic pancreatic tissue, arteriovenous fistula, and hemangioma, IOE is useful for intraoperative localization.

- Lack of DAE facility – DAE is available at most centers in developed countries. However, in low income countries or in limited resource setting, IOE is a safe and effective alternative to DAE. It allows diagnosis and treatment of the small bowel diseases in the same sitting.

3. Techniques

IOE is mainly performed via conventional laparotomy. However, it can be performed by mini-laparotomy [22, 23] or laparoscopy [24–27]. IOE can be performed by gastroscope, colonoscope, pediatric scope or balloon enteroscope depending upon the probable site of the lesions, the indication for IOE and the availability of the equipments. In rare circumstances, IOE can be performed using a laparoscope [28]. IOE can be conducted through oral route, anal route and through an enterotomy site (**Figure 7**). The choice of the preferred route for IOE depends upon the location of the lesion.

The patients are admitted before the procedure. All routine investigations including cardiorespiratory work up are done to rule out any contraindication for surgery. The day before the procedure the standard bowel preparation (the same as for colonoscopy) with either polyethylene glycol or sodium phosphate is given [29]. The patients are asked to fast for 6 hours before the surgery.

All the endoscopes and the accessories are sterilized before the procedure. The endoscopist has to scrub like any other member of the operating team. The part of the endoscope to be inserted in the operating field is covered with a plastic sleeve routinely used for laparoscopic procedures. This will help in maintaining the sterility of the procedure. The procedure is performed under general anesthesia.

3.1 Intraoperative endoscopy via oral route

- Transoral endoscopy can be performed with the patient in supine or left lateral position [30]. Prior to the insertion of the endoscope, a nasogastric tube is placed to decompress the stomach. Subsequently, the nasogastric tube is removed and the gastroscope is inserted.

- Like the routine endoscopy, the gastroscope is passed in to the duodenum (**Figure 7A**). If the intraoperative endoscopy is pre-planned, then the endoscope can be passed as far as possible into the duodenum before the abdominal incision to take benefit of the tamponade effect of the abdominal wall.

- During the passage of the endoscope, a loop tends to form along the greater curvature of the stomach and the 'C' of the duodenum. Once, the endoscope has reached the jejunum, the assistant surgeon can place the right hand along the greater curvature of the stomach and the left hand over the second part of the duodenum to straighten the endoscope. This will help in going further deep in to the small bowel via the oral route.

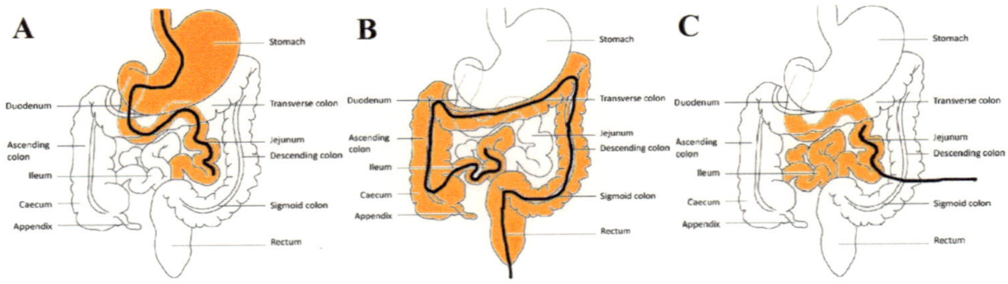

Figure 7.
Schematic presentation of different routes for intraoperative enteroscopy: (A) Transoral route, (B) transanal route and (C) enteroscopy via enterotomy.

- Deeper passage of the scope in to the jejunum is performed with the help of the operating team. Mobile small bowel and mesentery is necessary to facilitate smooth passage of the scope and avoid bowel injury. Hence, if adhesions are present then adhesiolysis should be performed by the operative team before initiating IOE.

- For the examination of the small bowel beyond the proximal jejunum, the operating surgeon straightens the bowel loops as the endoscopist gently pushes the endoscope in to the jejunum. Subsequently, about 40–50 cm of small bowel is telescoped on to the shaft of the endoscope by the operating surgeon.

- Advancement of the endoscope through the small bowel must be smooth, slow, gentle and under direct vision to avoid mucosal trauma by the endoscope and avoid excessive tension on the mesentery.

- The mucosa is thoroughly examined during the insertion and withdrawal of the endoscope. Any lesion if detected is biopsied or excised endoscopically using the standard techniques. Bleeding from the endoscopic excision site can be controlled by endoscopic techniques or transmural sutures by the operating team.

- If the lesion is big and requires surgical excision, then the site of the lesion must be marked with a simple suture by the operating team.

- In most cases, it is possible to examine the whole small bowel via oral route using the standard-length colonoscope. But if not possible, then the terminal ileum can be examined in a retrograde fashion via transanal route.

- The distal most point up to which the scope reaches in the small bowel is marked with a simple suture by the surgical team.

- Throughout the procedure, the operating room lights are dimmed so that the endoscopy team is able to clearly visualize the bowel mucosa and the location of the endoscope. The abnormal vascular lesions can be better identified by transillumination.

- During withdrawal, after inspecting the mucosa, the air is aspirated by the endoscopist and the surgeon occludes the intestinal lumen with his index and middle fingers to avoid re-insufflation.

- After completion of the endoscopy, the lesions at the marked sites are excised surgically by multiple enterotomies or segmental bowel resection depending upon the intraoperative findings.

3.2 IOE via anal route

- This is the least preferred route for IOE due to limited maneuverability.
- The procedure can be performed in lithotomy or left lateral position.
- The steps are similar to that of colonoscopy (**Figure 7B**). In case of difficulty in negotiating the scope across the colonic flexures, the operating surgeons can guide the scope.
- Small lesions can be excised or biopsied endoscopically while large lesions can be marked with simple suture for subsequent surgical excision.
- After reaching the ileocecal region, the surgeon slowly pushes the ileal loops over the scope for the mucosal examination. However, evaluation of the small bowel beyond terminal ileum via anal route is difficult.
- In such cases, if there is a large colonic lesion requiring surgical excision, a colotomy can be made near the site of resection and the colonoscope can be advanced through it to facilitate further small bowel examination.

3.3 IOE via enterotomy

- After appropriate adhesiolysis, whole of the small bowel is freed.
- A circular purse-string suture is taken at a suitable point (usually the mid portion) of the small intestine on the anti-mesenteric side [6]. A small enterotomy is made at the center of the purse string suture just sufficient enough to allow the passage of the endoscope.
- The endoscope is inserted through the enterotomy and the circular suture is tied around the scope over the bowel to prevent air leak during insufflation (**Figure 7C**).
- First, the proximal part of the small intestine is examined due to lower bacterial load.
- Enteroscopy should be performed slowly with gradual advancement of the scope and minimum insufflation to prevent bowel injury.
- Endoscopic biopsy or excision is performed for the visualized mucosa lesions as appropriate. If surgical excision is required, then the site of lesion is marked by the operating surgeon with a simple suture.
- During the inspection of the proximal half of the small bowel, the distal part if clamped and vice-versa to prevent over-inflation.
- The endoscopic views during IOE are different from the routine endoscopic picture due to transillumination by the operating lights in the theater. However, the operating lights can be dimmed if required as per the endoscopist's choice.

3.4 Insertion of port in bowel

- In order to avoid contamination of the operative field, some authors have described the use of laparoscopic port.
- In this technique, a 12-mm or 15-mm bladeless laparoscopic port with or without balloon is inserted from the enterotomy site in to the bowel [31–34].
- The laparoscopic camera sleeve is fixed to the port with tape.
- The endoscope is passed through the camera sleeve and port in to the bowel for enteroscopy.
- This technique allows to maintain the sterility of the operative field.

3.5 Laparoscopic assisted panenteroscopy

- In this technique, in order to avoid the laparotomy, the endoscope is passed through one of the 12- or 15-mm laparoscopic port [24–26].
- IOE can be performed via oral [25, 27, 34], anal [35] or enterotomy route [24, 26].
- The procedure for IOE via oral or anal route is same as described above except that the adhesiolysis and handling of the small bowel is performed laparoscopically. Additionally, the bowel insufflation has to be minimum to allow space for laparoscopic bowel manipulation [24].
- For IOE through enterotomy, a small jejunotomy is made and the endoscope is passed through it in to the bowel.
- Although the mobility of the scope is restricted compared to conventional IOE through laparotomy, it is possible to visualize the whole small intestine with careful manipulation of the small bowel loops.
- After the withdrawal of the endoscope, the enterotomy wound is sutured laparoscopically.
- However, this procedure is technically more demanding and time consuming. Both the laparoscopist and endoscopist need to be highly skilled and experienced.

3.6 Single incision laparoscopic (SILS) assisted enteroscopy

- DAE is possible in most of the cases. However, in some cases, DAE may be difficult due to previous laparotomy, or inability to reduce the forming loops during DAE leading to incomplete bowel examination.
- In such cases, DAE can be performed under laparoscopic guidance. Laparoscopy can be undertaken by conventional 3-ports or SILS technique [21, 27].

- In SILS technique, a SILS port is inserted at the umbilicus. A 10-mm laparoscope and two 5-mm non-traumatic graspers are inserted through the SILS port. Laparoscopic adhesiolysis is performed before starting enteroscopy.

- Enteroscopy is performed using conventional flexible endoscope or DBE. Surgical manipulation of the bowel loops is done during enteroscopy if required.

- The visualized lesions can be excised endoscopically or laparoscopically depending upon the location and size of the lesions and the available expertise.

- In a recent study of 13 patients who underwent SILS enteroscopy, target pathology could be reached in all but one patient with PJS, in whom antegrade DBE failed to reach up to the target polyp and a small enterotomy was required to complete IOE and excise the polyp [21].

4. Outcomes

A review of 16 studies involving 468 patients by Voron T, et al. reported that the site of bleeding could be successfully identified in 371 patients (79.3%) [16]. The predominant lesions responsible for obscure GI bleed were vascular lesions (n = 227, 61%), benign ulcers (n = 70, 19%), tumors (n = 36, 10%) and diverticula (n = 15, 4%) [16]. The most common route of IOE was transoral followed by trans-enterotomy. A recent study by Manatsathit W, et al. also reported vascular lesions, ulcers and tumors to be the most common lesions detected on IOE [36].

The reported rates of diagnostic and therapeutic yield of IOE are 79.3% (58–100%) and 75.7% (48–94%), respectively [1–10, 16, 36]. The diagnostic yield for obscure GI bleeding after non-diagnostic abdominal imaging has been reported to be 91–100% and after non-diagnostic VCE/DAE varies from 14.2% to 66.7% [1, 6, 9, 36]. Traditionally, the treatment of the lesions detected during IOE were performed surgically. But, with the advancement in the endoscopic techniques, the lesions are being increasingly tackled endoscopically as far as possible and surgical treatment is performed for the rest of the lesions especially in condition like PJS.

5. Complications

IOE via enterotomy converts clean surgery in to clean-contaminated surgery which increases the risk of infective complications. Another problem of IOE is excessive bowel handling which increases the risk of postoperative ileus. The reported complication rates of IOE vary between 1 and 50% [16, 36, 37]. According to a combined data of 10 studies involving 309 patients, the overall morbidity rate was 16.8% which included surgical and medical morbidities [37]. The complications were mainly related to general anesthesia, laparotomy and bowel surgery required for bowel lesions and not solely related to IOE. Prolonged postoperative ileus was one of the predominant surgical morbidity. Other morbidities included bowel obstruction, wound infection, intrabdominal collections/abscess, intra-abdominal bleeding, chest infection and cardiorespiratory failure [18, 37]. The complications directly related to IOE include mucosal laceration, bowel wall hematoma, mesenteric hematoma or bleeding due to excessive handling during IOE and rarely, bowel perforation [38].

The overall mortality rate of IOE from the combined data of 14 studies including 419 patients was 5% [37]. The main causes of death were multiorgan failure, septic shock, diffuse intravascular coagulopathy and hemorrhagic shock [37].

An important issue in patients with obscure GI bleed after any investigation or treatment is the development of recurrent GI bleed. The reported incidence of recurrent GI bleed ranges from 13–52% in different series [9, 36, 37]. It is important to note that differentiation between iatrogenic mucosal trauma from mucosal vascular lesions by IOE is difficult [39]. Secondly, vascular lesions can be evanescent, hence early IOE or at time of bleeding can make the detection of these lesions possible [40]. Other reasons for rebleeding could be appearance of new lesions due to same or different disease, incomplete endoscopic treatment of the existing lesions such as angiodysplasia, etc.

6. Limitations

IOE involves lot of small bowel handling and manipulation to allow smooth passage of the endoscopy across the bowel loops. In cases of dense adhesions with shortened mesentery, IOE can be difficult and increase the risk of bowel injury. Another situation where IOE is difficult is in the presence of massive GI bleeding as the lumen is completely filled with blood and examination of the bowel mucosa is not possible [7].

7. Conclusions

With the increasing use of DAE, the need for IOE has reduced. However, it continues to be an extremely useful tool in patients with obscure GI bleed, multiple polyposis syndromes, multiple foreign bodies or bowel obstruction where DAE cannot be performed or has failed. Moreover, IOE has been found to reduce the need for repeated surgeries by allowing complete small bowel examination and treatment in the same sitting. Although IOE via laparotomy remains the gold standard, availability of advanced minimally invasive equipments have allowed IOE to be performed via multiport or single port laparoscopy.

Conflict of interest

The authors have no conflict of interest to declare.

Author details

Rahul Gupta[1*], Arvind K. Singh[2], Jyoti Gupta[3] and Houssem Ammar[4]

1 Department of Gastrointestinal Surgery, Synergy Institute of Medical Sciences, Dehradun, India

2 Department of Gastroenterology, Synergy Institute of Medical Sciences, Dehradun, India

3 Department of Radiation Oncology, Swami Rama Himalayan University, Dehradun, India

4 Department of Surgery, Sousse Hospital, Sousse, Tunisia

*Address all correspondence to: rahul.g.85@gmail.com

IntechOpen

© 2021 The Author(s). Licensee IntechOpen. This chapter is distributed under the terms of the Creative Commons Attribution License (http://creativecommons.org/licenses/by/3.0), which permits unrestricted use, distribution, and reproduction in any medium, provided the original work is properly cited.

References

[1] Hartmann D, Schmidt H, Bolz G, Schilling D, Kinzel F, Eickhoff A, et al. A prospective two-center study comparing wireless capsule endoscopy with intraoperative enteroscopy in patients with obscure GI bleeding. Gastrointest Endosc. 2005;61:826-832.

[2] Zaman A, Sheppard B, Katon RM. Total peroral intraoperative enteroscopy for obscure GI bleeding using a dedicated push enteroscope: diagnostic yield and patient outcome. Gastrointest Endosc. 1999;50:506-10.

[3] Douard R, Wind P, Panis Y, Marteau P, Bouhnik Y, Cellier C, et al. Intraoperative enteroscopy for diagnosis and management of unexplained gastrointestinal bleeding. Am J Surg. 2000;180:181-4.

[4] Kendrick ML, Buttar NS, Anderson MA, Lutzke LS, Peia D, Wang KK, et al. Contribution of intraoperative enteroscopy in the management of obscure gastrointestinal bleeding. J Gastrointest Surg. 2001;5:162-7.

[5] Jakobs R, Hartmann D, Benz C, Shilling D, Weickert U, Eickhoff A, et al. Diagnosis of obscure gastrointestinal bleeding by intra-operative enteroscopy in 81 consecutive patients. World J Gastroenterol. 2006;12:313-6.

[6] Kopácová M, Bures J, Vykouril L, Hladík P, Simkovic D, Jon B, et al. Intraoperative enteroscopy: ten years' experience at a single tertiary center. Surg Endosc. 2007;21:1111-6.

[7] Schulz HJ, Schmidt H. Intraoperative enteroscopy. Gastrointest Endosc Clin N Am. 2009;19:371-9.

[8] Douard R, Wind P, Berger A, Maniere T, Landi B, Cellier C, et al. Role of intraoperative enteroscopy in the management of obscure gastrointestinal bleeding at the time of video-capsule endoscopy. Am J Surg. 2009;198:6-11.

[9] Monsanto P, Almeida N, Lérias C, Figueiredo P, Gouveia H, Sofia C. Is there still a role for intraoperative enteroscopy in patients with obscure gastrointestinal bleeding? Rev Esp Enferm Dig. 2012;104:190-6.

[10] Green J, Schlieve CR, Friedrich AK, Baratta K, Ma DH, Min M, et al. Approach to the diagnostic workup and management of small bowel lesions at a tertiary care center. J Gastointest Surg. 2018;22:1034-1042.

[11] Pennazio M. Enteroscopy in the diagnosis and management of obscure gastrointestinal bleeding. Gastrointest Endosc Clin N Am. 2009;19:409-26.

[12] Ell C, May A. Mid-gastrointestinal bleeding: capsule endoscopy and push-and-pull enteroscopy give rise to a new medical term. Endoscopy 2006;38:73-5.

[13] Beggs AD, Latchford AR, Vasen HF, Moslein G, Alonso A, Aretz S, et al. Peutz-Jeghers syndrome: a systematic review and recommendations for management. Gut. 2010; 59: 975-986.

[14] Perrod G, Samaha E, Perez-Cuadrado-Robles E, Berger A, Benosman H, Khater S, et al. Small bowel polyp resection using device-assisted enteroscopy in Peutz-Jeghers syndrome: Results of a specialized tertiary care centre. United European Gastroenterol J. 2020;8:204-210.

[15] Lee DH, Shin HD, Cho WH, Shin KH, Lee S, Shin JE, et al. Polyp Clearance via Operative and Endoscopic Polypectomy in Patients With Peutz-Jeghers Syndrome After Multiple Small Bowel Resections. Intest Res. 2014; 12:320-327.

[16] Voron T, Rahmi G, Bonnet S, Malamut G, Wind P, Cellier C, et al. Intraoperative endoscopy Is there still a role? Gastrointest Endosc Clin N Am. 2017;27:153-170.

[17] Hotokezaka M, Jimi SI, Hidaka H, Eto TA, Chijiiwa K. Intraoperative enteroscopy in minimally invasive surgery. Surg Laparosc Endosc Percutan Tech. 2007;17:492-4.

[18] Hotokezaka M, Jimi SI, Hidaka H, Maehara N, Eto TA, Chijiiwa K. Role of intraoperative enteroscopy for surgical decision making with Crohn's disease. Surg Endosc. 2007;21:1238-42.

[19] Gupta R, Singh AK, Ammar H. Colonic obstruction: a rare complication of acute pancreatitis. ANZ J Surg. 2020;90:E141-E142.

[20] Kulkarni VM, Gandhi JA, Gupta RA, Deokar RB, Karnik ND, Nadkar MY. Body packer syndrome. J Postgrad Med. 2012;58:225-6.

[21] Stasinos I, Kamperidis N, Murino A, Jenkins JT, Warusavitarne J, Fraser C, Humphries A. Single incision laparoscopic assisted double balloon enteroscopy: a novel technique to manage small bowel pathology. Surg Endosc. 2020;34:2773-2779.

[22] Matsushita M, Hajiro K, Takakuwa H, Fuhikawa T. Laparoscopicallyassistedpanenteroscopy for gastrointestinal bleeding of obscure origin. Gastrointest Endosc. 1997;46:474-5.

[23] Chui CH, Jacobsen AS. Transumbilical approach to intraoperative enteroscopy in a child with intussusception and Peutz-Jeghers syndrome. J Laparosc Adv Surg Tech. 2006;16:543-5.

[24] Reddy ND, Rao VG. Laparoscopically assisted panenteroscopy for snare excision. Gastrointest Endosc. 1996;44:208-9.

[25] Ingrosso M, Prete F, Pisani A, Carbonara R, Azzarone A, Francavilla A. Laparoscopically assisted total enteroscopy: a new approach to small intestinal diseases. Gastrointest Endosc. 1999;49:651-3.

[26] Sriram PV, Rao GV, Reddy DN. Laparoscopically assisted panenteroscopy. Gastrointest Endosc. 2001;54:805-6.

[27] Ross AS, Dye C, Prachand VN. Laparoscopic-assisted double-balloon enteroscopy for small-bowel polyp surveillance and treatment in patients with Peutz-Jeghers syndrome. Gastrointest Endosc. 2006;64:984-8.

[28] Agarwal A. Use of the laparoscope to perform intraoperative enteroscopy. Surg Endosc. 1999;13:1143-4.

[29] Kopácová M, Bures J, Ferko A, Tachecí I, Rejchrt S. Comparison of intraoperative enteroscopy and double-balloon enteroscopy for the diagnosis and treatment of Peutz-Jeghers syndrome. Surg Endosc. 2010;24:1904-10.

[30] Bowden TA Jr. Endoscopy of the small intestine. Surg Clin North Am. 1989;69:1237-47.

[31] Gorski YC, Gorski TF, Chung HJ, Genato R. A new technique for intraoperative enteroscopy using a 12-mm trocar. Surg Endosc. 1999;13:724-726.

[32] Tartaglia D, Mazzoni A, Puglisi AG, Coccolini F, Chiarugi M. Intra-operative enteroscopy for the identification of obscure bleeding source caused by gastrointestinal angiodysplasias: through a balloon-tip trocar is better. Colorectal Dis. 2020 Sep 3. Doi: 10.1111/codi.15348. Online ahead of print.

[33] Smyth R, Richardson C. A method for performing intraoperative enteroscopy. Ann R Coll Surg Engl. 2017;99:178.

[34] Pontane S, Pironi D, Arcieri S, Eberspacher C, Panarese A, Filippini A. Intraoperative enteroscopy by standard colonoscope with a minimal contamination technique. Surg Laparosc Endosc Percutan Tech. 2013;23:e11-3.

[35] Meister TE, Nicki NJ, Park A. Laparoscopic-assisted panenteroscopy. Gastrointest Endosc. 2001;53:236-9.

[36] Manatsathit W, Khruchareon U, Jensen DM, Hines OJ, Kovacs T, Ohning G, et al. Laparotomy and intraoperative enteroscopy for obscure gastrointestinal bleeding before and after the era of video capsule endoscopy and deep enteroscopy: a tertiary center experience. Am J Surg. 2018;215:603-609.

[37] Bonnet S, Douard R, Malamut G, Cellier C, Wind P. Intraoperative enteroscopy in the management of obscure gastrointestinal Bleeding. Dig Liver Dis. 2013;45:277-284.

[38] Krisham RS, Kent RB III. Enterovaginal fistula as a complication of intraoperative small bowel endoscopy. Surg Laparosc Endosc. 1998;8:388-9.

[39] Goldstein JL, Eisen GM, Lewis B, Gralnek IM, Aisenberg J, Bhadra P, et al. Small bowel mucosal injury is reduced in healthy subjects treated with celecoxib compared with ibuprofen plus omeprazole, as assessed by video capsule endoscopy. Aliment Pharmacol Ther. 2007;25:1211-22.

[40] Gerson LB. Outcomes associated with deep enteroscopy. Gastrointest Endosc Clin N Am. 2009;19:481-96.

Section 6

Small Bowel Perforation

Chapter 7

Early Recognition and Management of Small Bowel Perforation

Md. Yusuf Afaque, Noha Rehman, S. Amjad Ali Rizvi and Meraj Ahmed

Abstract

Enteroscopy has a procedure-related perforation rate from less than 1% to 6.5%. It seems to be higher in therapeutic enteroscopy, especially polypectomy of large polyps, and in patients who have altered surgical anatomy. Early recognition is life-saving and studies have shown that if surgery is done within 12 hours of perforation the prognosis is better. In a patient who has undergone small bowel endoscopy the diagnosis of small bowel perforation should be suspected if the patient has acute pain in the abdomen. Early diagnosis should be the goal with prompt surgical correction.

Keywords: small bowel perforation, peritonitis, laparoscopy, enteroscopy, small bowel endoscopy

1. Introduction

Enteroscopy has a procedure-related perforation rate from less than 1% to 6.5% [1–3]. It seems to be higher in therapeutic enteroscopy, especially polypectomy of large polyps, and in patients with altered surgical anatomy. Early recognition is life-saving and surgery performed within 12 hours carries a better prognosis. It was seen in peptic perforations that a delay of more than 24 hours increased mortality seven to eight times, complication rate to three times, and length of hospital stay to two times, compared with a delay of 6 hours or less [4]. Early diagnosis should be the goal followed by prompt surgical correction.

2. Bowel pathologies that increase the risk of perforation during small bowel endoscopy/enteroscopy

Bowel pathologies with increased susceptibility for perforation during small bowel endoscopy include – Crohn's disease, anastomotic stricture, radiation stricture, altered surgical anatomy (ileoanal, ileocolic anastomosis), and intestinal lymphoma. The perforation rate during double balloon enteroscopy is seen more with the retrograde technique compared to anterograde [5]. Also, more perforations are seen with therapeutic procedures like polypectomy of large polyp (> 3 cm), argon plasma coagulation for AV malformations, and dilations of small bowel strictures [3, 5, 6]. Furthermore, endoscopy associated perforations are more in patients with inflammatory bowel disease (IBD) as compared to non-IBD patients, with disease severity and steroid use being the two of the strong predictors for perforation [7–10]. In a systematic review, the total rate of perforation with enteroscopy in Crohn's disease was 4.27 per 1000 procedures (diagnostic and therapeutic procedures) and it was nearly 4 times that of diagnostic balloon assisted enteroscopy for all indications (1.1 per 1000 procedures) [11].

3. Early recognition of perforation by simple bedside examination

In a patient who has undergone small bowel endoscopy the diagnosis of small bowel perforation should be suspected if the patient has acute pain in the abdomen. The severity of pain will progressively increase. The patient will lie still as any movement will exacerbate the pain. Even the respiration will be shallow for this reason. This differentiates it from other acute pathologies like acute pancreatitis in which the patient is restless and changes posture to find relief. The physical examination will reveal a sick look, tachycardia, and features of dehydration along with the signs of peritonitis. Perforation causes third space loss of body fluid. This along with bacteremia and systemic inflammatory response leads to hypotension and decreased urine output. The abdomen will be very tender and guarding will be present. A board-like rigidity may be felt. Loss of liver dullness on percussion will further confirm the presence of free air in the peritoneal cavity. Bowel sounds will be absent due to paralytic ileus caused by peritonitis. After 4–6 hours of perforation (gastro-duodenal perforation), the peritoneal cavity acid becomes diluted and there is a decrease in pain and guarding. It may seem that the patient is improving but, in reality, is deteriorating [12].

Making the diagnosis of perforation may be difficult in the early period because of subtle signs and symptoms. The classical peritoneal signs may fail to elicit in a morbidly obese patient. Thus a high index of suspicion should be kept in mind for patients complaining of undue pain following endoscopy. Any patient with difficult endoscopy should have close post procedure monitoring for early detection of complications. Tachycardia, dehydration, or decreased urine output should alarm the clinician. Repeated abdominal examination can detect any new abdominal signs. Lessons can be learnt from trauma surgery. In a hemodynamically stable patient with an anterior abdominal stab wound with the peritoneal breach, serial abdominal examination is a standard technique for picking the peritonitis early.

4. Role of basic laboratory investigation like TLC and serum lactate in early diagnosis

Laboratory workup will confirm the diagnosis of small bowel perforation apart from a careful history and physical examination. It is particularly helpful in elderly or seriously ill patients in whom signs and symptoms are less reliable. An elevated (>12,000/ cumm) or decreased white blood cells (< 4000/cumm) confirms inflammation or infection [13]. If TLC is normal, an increase in the number of neutrophils in differential counts or bandemia (> 10% band forms) is indicative of infection. The hemoglobin level will help in deciding the blood transfusion requirement. Serum electrolytes, blood urea nitrogen and, serum creatinine measurements will provide information about the fluid losses associated with third space loss, vomiting, delayed presentation, etc. Lactate level serves as a surrogate marker for tissue perfusion and correlates with anaerobic metabolism. A raised lactate level indicates bowel ischemia, shock, and sepsis. Lactate levels have been more specific than leukocyte count in diagnosing abdominal sepsis [14]. However, lactate levels can also be elevated in hepatic failure, dehydration, and drug abuse. Metabolic acidosis will be present in sepsis. Coagulation profiles such as platelet count, prothrombin time, international normalized ratio, etc. are important in the preoperative assessment of patients with liver disease or those on anticoagulants. These may also be deranged due to sepsis. Other biochemical markers of inflammation include C-reactive protein and pro-calcitonin which when used in adjunct with complete blood count and other clinical signs help in making the diagnosis, assessing severity and prognosis, and guiding treatment.

5. Role of X-ray abdomen and CT scan in confirming the diagnosis

Plain radiography remains the most frequently ordered examination in patients with suspected perforation. Pneumoperitoneum is present in the rupture of any hollow viscous. It may also be observed following recent abdominal surgery, paracentesis, and pneumatosis intestinalis. Benign pneumoperitoneum may rarely develop following endoscopy due to transmural passage of insufflated air without bowel perforation [15]. Plain radiography can detect about 55–85% of patients with pneumoperitoneum [16]. It can detect as little as 1–2 ml of free air [17]. Upright lateral chest radiograph has better sensitivity than upright postero-anterior chest radiograph [18]. Upright positions including left lateral decubitus are uncomfortable in critically ill patients in the emergency setting. In such patients supine decubitus anteroposterior view of the thorax and anteroposterior or lateral view of the abdomen are generally requested [19].

Free air can be visualized in different shapes, sizes, and locations in the abdominal cavity. On upright postero-anterior chest or abdominal radiography, free air is visualized as a translucent crescent below the diaphragm (**Figure 1**). These free-air signs can be categorized as bowel-related, right-upper-quadrant, peritoneal ligament- related, or other signs [20]. Rigler sign is the visualization of both sides of the bowel wall in a supine abdominal radiograph (**Figure 2**). The presence of normal gas

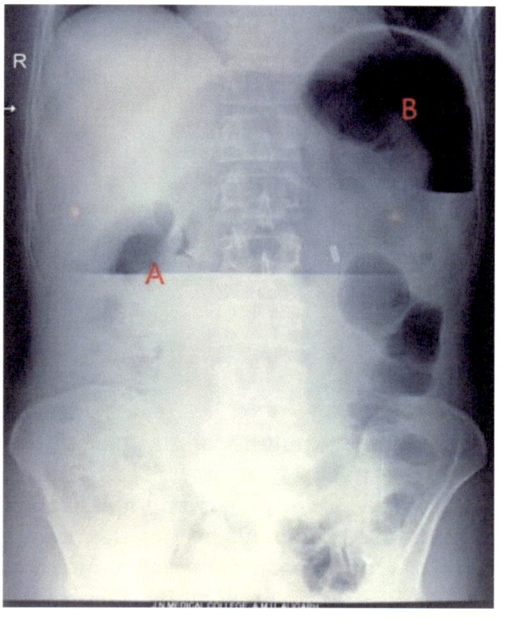

Figure 1.
X-ray abdomen showing A-Giant pneumoperitoneum appearing as an air-fluid level in the peritoneal cavity. B-pneumoperitoneum on the left side may be confused with fundal gas.

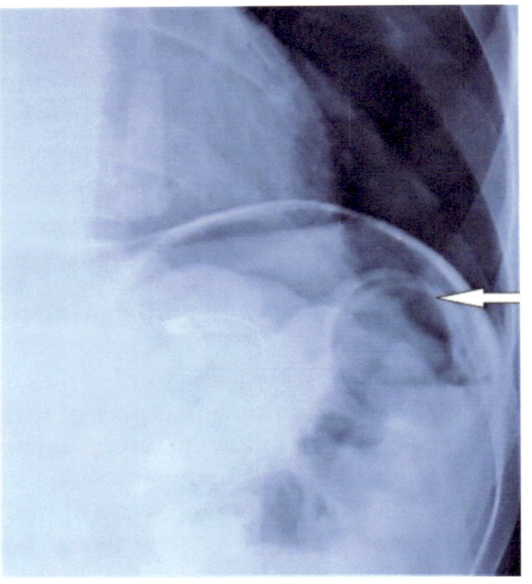

Figure 2.
Rigler sign.

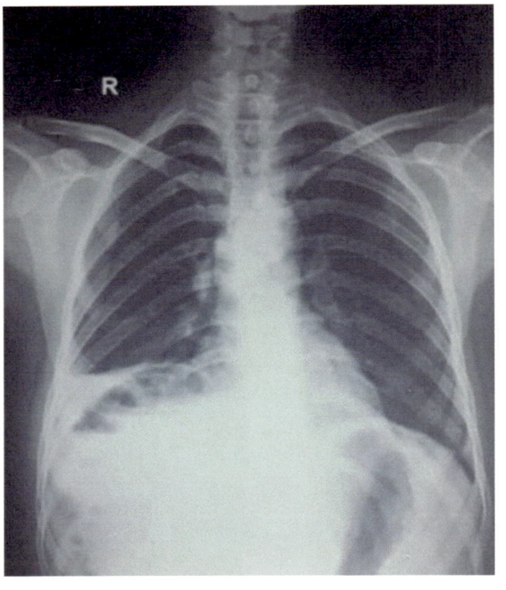

Figure 3.
X-ray chest showing Chilaiditi sign.

in the bowel lumen, as well as free extraluminal gas, makes the bowel wall outline nicely visible. It is seen when a large quantity of free gas is present in the abdomen. Hyperlucent liver sign is also seen in a supine radiograph. Intraperitoneal free air may outline the various peritoneal ligaments making them visible along their course giving rise to various signs: falciform ligament sign, ligamentum teres sign, "inverted V" sign, urachus sign, etc. [20]. Along with it air in the subcutaneous tissue can also be visualized. Pneumoperitoneum is often absent in the perforation of the retroperitoneal duodenum. A confusing picture related to pneumoperitoneum is the Chilaiditi sign. It is the interposition of the bowel, commonly colon, between the right hemidiaphragm and the liver. It can be falsely diagnosed as pneumoperitoneum. Features that are suggestive of Chilaiditi sign are gas between liver and diaphragm and haustra in the gas suggesting that it is bowel and not free air (**Figure 3**) [21].

Although plain radiography is good modality in suspected cases of hollow viscus perforation, ultrasonography can be helpful in certain scenarios because of the absence of radiation exposure, bedside availability, no pre-procedural preparation, and speed. It can be used in pregnant females and sick patients. It can detect free fluid in the abdomen and rule out other causes of acute abdominal pain. It may not help in the early period of perforation when the amount of free fluid is scant for detection.

Computed tomography (CT) scan is very sensitive and specific for perforation of the gastrointestinal tract (80–100%) [22]. It is more sensitive than plain radiography for small or retroperitoneal perforations. In addition to free air, it can also detect the location and size of perforation and any fluid collection. Direct CT signs of intestinal perforation are free gas and extra-luminal leak of oral contrast (**Figure 4**) [23]. Indirect signs include misty mesentery, fluid collection, bowel wall thickening, and extra-luminal fecal matter [24]. In a prospective study of 85 patients, the MDCT images confirmed the site of gastrointestinal tract perforation in 73 (86%) patients.

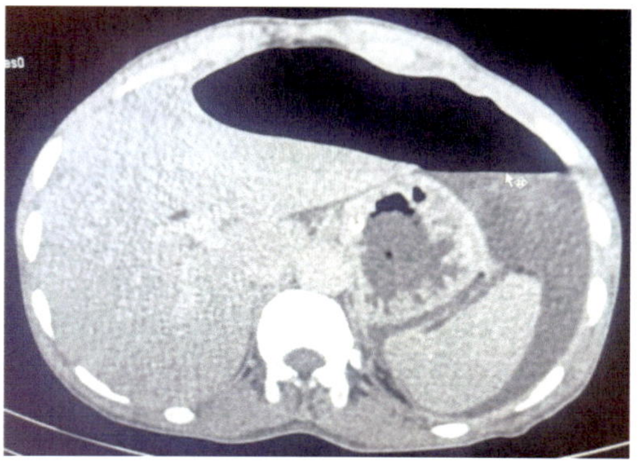

Figure 4.
CECT abdomen showing big pneumoperitoneum anteriorly and left side intra-abdominal collection. Same patient as shown in **Figure 1.**

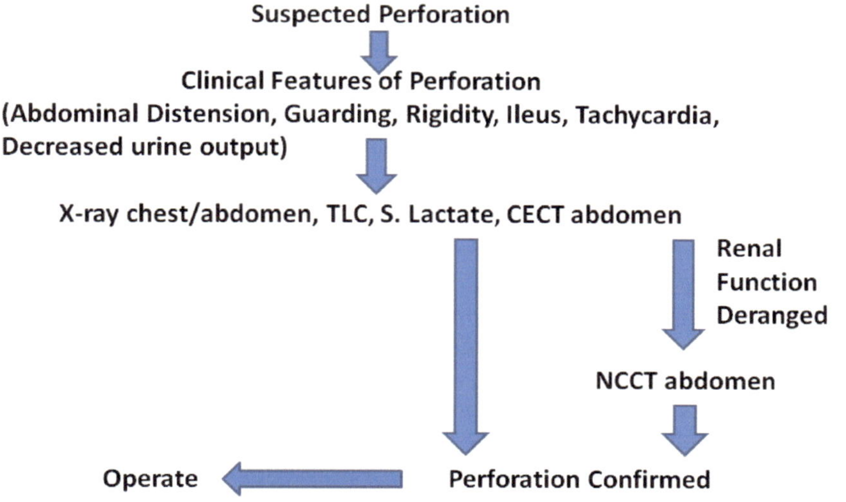

Figure 5.
Flowchart for the diagnosis of small bowel perforation.

Furthermore, the logistic regression showed that extra-luminal air, segmental bowel wall thickening, and focal defect of the intestinal wall were strong predictors of the site of perforation [25].

Signs present in plain radiography are also seen in scout view in CT. When contrast is contraindicated, then even plain CT is of help, in diagnosing perforation. The European Society of Gastrointestinal Endoscopy (ESGE) recommends that clinical features suggestive of perforation after an endoscopy should be rapidly and carefully evaluated and documented with a CT scan [26]. See flowchart for the diagnosis of intestinal perforation (**Figure 5**).

6. Resuscitation, supportive measures, and preparation for surgery

Evaluation and resuscitation should go hand in hand. The intravascular fluid deficit should be corrected considering systemic diseases in acutely ill patients. Warmed crystalloids (normal saline or lactated Ringer solution) should be started using wide-bore IV cannula. Fluid therapy should be guided according to physical signs (pulse rate, blood pressure), urine output, lactate levels, CVP, etc. Patients who are not responsive to adequate fluid therapy should be started on vasopressors. Nasogastric tube insertion prevents aspiration in patients with altered mental status and the elderly. Foley's catheterization is needed to measure urine output.

Parenteral analgesics (tramadol, paracetamol, NSAID, etc) should be started in an adequate dose in combination, keeping in mind the renal function of the patient. We generally avoid diclofenac in bowel repair as animal studies have shown an increased risk of post-surgery leak [27]. Broad-spectrum antibiotic therapy (piperacillin + tazobactum or meropenem, etc. along with metronidazole) should be started to control on-going sepsis. The antibiotics can later be continued as indicated or changed according to culture and sensitivity.

The anesthetic evaluation would include the American Society of Anesthesiologists (ASA) classification system to stratify patients according to the degree of perioperative risks [28]. Thromboprophylaxis should be started in high-risk patients that include mechanical devices (thromboembolic deterrent stocking and pneumatic compression boots) and drugs (heparin and LMWH) [29]. Risk factors for deep vein thrombosis include increased age, obesity, chronic diseases (diabetes, COPD, malignancy), corticosteroid therapy, and past or family history of thromboembolic disease. Written consent for surgery is taken and the patient and the family should be explained about the possibility of multiple staged surgeries, temporary stomas, postoperative ICU care, and expected complications of surgery.

7. The indication of laparoscopy in the diagnosis and management of intestinal perforation

Laparoscopy has a role in the diagnosis of perforations that are sometimes not detected by imaging tools. It allows complete visualization and exploration of the abdominal cavity. Laparoscopy is considered safe and a valid diagnostic tool and has a diagnostic benefit of 89–100% in the acute abdomen [30]. However, in cases of small bowel perforation, it is more of a therapeutic modality. Patients treated with laparoscopy have smaller incisions (**Figure 6**), reduced post-operative pain, early return of bowel movements, shorter hospital stay, and faster return to normal activity. Various factors limit the role of laparoscopy in patients with perforation peritonitis. Respiratory and hemodynamic stability is necessary before performing laparoscopy. Pneumoperitoneum affects the respiratory and cardiovascular parameters, thus patients with comorbidities

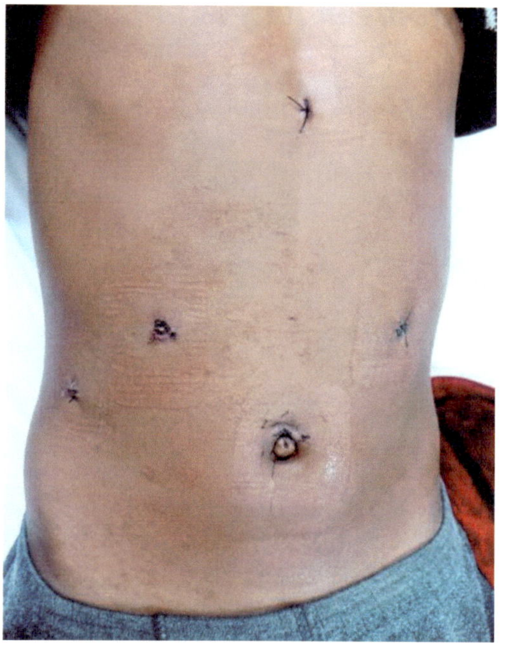

Figure 6.
Small incisions of laparoscopic surgery.

should be properly evaluated before the procedure. The presence of dense intra-abdominal adhesions and the expertise of the surgeon are other parameters that affect the feasibility of laparoscopic procedure [30, 31].

The choice of bowel repair technique depends upon the condition of the patient as well as the bowel. Primary suture repair can be done for small perforation. Resection of the involved bowel with anastomosis is required if the surrounding bowel is unhealthy or the perforation is large (more than 50% of the bowel circumference). The primary repair/anastomosis is at risk in conditions that impair healing. An obstructed, irradiated, inflamed, or ischemic intestine is traditionally considered high risk. Other than this, systemic factors like malnutrition, hypotension, diabetes, renal failure, chronic liver disease, anemia, steroid use, and other conditions causing immunocompromise lead to an increased risk of anastomotic failure [32]. If there are multiple risk factors for anastomotic leak then exteriorization of the perforated bowel as a stoma may be a safer option. It is followed by stoma closure after two to three months. However, in proximal jejunum, a stoma will lead to serious nutritional loss and if possible should be avoided. Complete lavage of all the abdominal recesses must always be done to prevent post-operative intra-abdominal collection (tertiary peritonitis). The patients have a good recovery after a timely repair.

8. Conclusion

In a patient who has undergone small bowel endoscopy the diagnosis of small bowel perforation should be suspected if the patient is presenting with an acute pain abdomen, especially after a therapeutic procedure.

The physical examination will reveal a sick look, tachycardia, and features of dehydration along with the abdominal signs of peritonitis.

Perforation is confirmed by x-ray abdomen, leucocytosis, and an increase in serum lactate. Computed tomography scan is very sensitive and specific for perforation of the gastrointestinal tract.

Early diagnosis should be the goal with prompt surgical correction, and the patients have a good recovery after timely repair.

Author details

Md. Yusuf Afaque*, Noha Rehman, S. Amjad Ali Rizvi and Meraj Ahmed
Department of Surgery, Jawaharlal Nehru Medical College and Hospital, Aligarh Muslim University, Aligarh, India

*Address all correspondence to: yusufafaque@gmail.com

IntechOpen

© 2021 The Author(s). Licensee IntechOpen. This chapter is distributed under the terms of the Creative Commons Attribution License (http://creativecommons.org/licenses/by/3.0), which permits unrestricted use, distribution, and reproduction in any medium, provided the original work is properly cited.

References

[1] Gerson LB. Capsule endoscopy and deep enteroscopy. Gastrointest Endosc. 2013;78(3):439-43.

[2] May A, Nachbar L, Pohl J, Ell C. Endoscopic interventions in the small bowel using double balloon enteroscopy: Feasibility and limitations. Am J Gastroenterol. 2007;102(3):527-35.

[3] Gerson LB, Tokar J, Chiorean M, Lo S, Decker GA, Cave D, et al. Complications Associated With Double Balloon Enteroscopy at Nine US Centers. Clin Gastroenterol Hepatol. 2009;7(11).

[4] Svanes C, Lie RT, Svanes K, Lie SA, Søreide O. Adverse effects of delayed treatment for perforated peptic ulcer. Ann Surg. 1994;220(2):168-75.

[5] Teshima CW, May G. Small bowel enteroscopy. Can J Gastroenterol. 2012;26(5):269-75.

[6] Mensink PBF, Haringsma J, Kucharzik T, Cellier C, Pérez-Cuadrado E, Mönkemüller K, et al. Complications of double balloon enteroscopy: A multicenter survey. Endoscopy. 2007;39(7):613-5.

[7] Mukewar S, Costedio M, Wu X, Bajaj N, Lopez R, Brzezinski A, et al. Severe adverse outcomes of endoscopic perforations in patients with and without IBD. Inflamm Bowel Dis. 2014;20(11):2056-66.

[8] Navaneethan U, Kochhar G, Phull H, Venkatesh PGK, Remzi FH, Kiran RP, et al. Severe disease on endoscopy and steroid use increase the risk for bowel perforation during colonoscopy in inflammatory bowel disease patients. J Crohn's Colitis. 2012;6(4):470-5.

[9] Navaneethan U, Parasa S, Venkatesh PGK, Trikudanathan G, Shen B. Prevalence and risk factors for colonic perforation during colonoscopy in hospitalized inflammatory bowel disease patients. J Crohn's Colitis. 2011;5(3):189-95.

[10] Odagiri H, Matsui H, Fushimi K, Kaise M, Yasunaga H. Factors associated with perforation related to diagnostic balloon-assisted enteroscopy: Analysis of a national inpatient database in Japan. Endoscopy. 2014;39(2).

[11] Arulanandan A, Dulai PS, Singh S, Sandborn WJ, Kalmaz D. Systematic review: Safety of balloon assisted enteroscopy in Crohn's disease. World J Gastroenterol. 2016;22(40):8999-9011.

[12] Lowry J. Browse's Introduction to the Symptoms and Signs of Surgical Disease (4th edn). Vol. 88, Annals of The Royal College of Surgeons of England. Royal College of Surgeons of England; 2006. 333 p.

[13] Dugar S, Choudhary C, Duggal A. Sepsis and septic shock: Guideline-based management. Cleve Clin J Med. 2020;87(1):53-64.

[14] Demircan M, Caglayan F, Deysine M, Fath JJ. Plasma D-lactate level: A useful marker to distinguish a perforated appendix from acute simple appendicitis. J Investig Surg. 2004;17(3):173-8.

[15] Ustek S, Boran M, Kismet K. Benign pneumoperitoneum after colonoscopy. Case Rep Med. 2010;2010.

[16] Roh JJ, Thompson JS, Harned RK, Hodgson PE. Value of pneumoperitoneum in the diagnosis of visceral perforation. Am J Surg. 1983;146(6):830-3.

[17] Hokama A, Nakamura M, Kobashigawa C, Chinen H, Kishir Nakamoto M, et al. Gastrointesti Signs of pneumoperitoneum. J Gastroenterol Hepatol. 2009;2

[18] Woodring JH, Heiser MJ. Detection of pneumoperitoneum on chest radiographs: Comparison of upright lateral and posteroanterior projections. Am J Roentgenol. 1995;165(1):45-7.

[19] Grassi R, Romano S, Pinto A, Romano L. Gastro-duodenal perforations: Conventional plain film, US and CT findings in 166 consecutive patients. Eur J Radiol. 2004;50(1):30-6.

[20] Pinto A, Miele V, Laura Schillirò M, Nasuto M, Chiaese V, Romano L, et al. Spectrum of Signs of Pneumoperitoneum. Semin Ultrasound, CT MRI. 2016;37(1):3-9.

[21] Chilaiditi D. Zur Frage der Hepatoptose und Ptose im allgemeinen im Anschluss an drei Falle von temporarer, partieller Leberverlagerung. Fortschr Rontgenstr. 1910;16:173-207.

[22] Cadenas Rodríguez L, Martí de Gracia M, Saturio Galán N, Pérez Dueñas V, Salvatierra Arrieta L, Garzón Moll G. Use of Multidetector Computed Tomography for Locating the Site of Gastrointestinal Tract Perforations. Cirugía Española (English Ed. 2013 May 1;91(5):316-23.

[23] Lo Re G, Mantia F La, Picone D, Salerno S, Vernuccio F, Midiri M. Small Bowel Perforations: What the Radiologist Needs to Know. Semin Ultrasound, CT MRI. 016;37(1):23-30.

into A, Scaglione M, Pinto F, no L, Grassi R, Rotondo A. Helical ed tomography diagnosis ntestinal perforation in patient. Emerg Radiol. 9-62.

Agneessens E, aertelaer V, Rubesova E, ccuracy of MDCT astrointestinal Roentgenol.

[26] Paspatis GA, Arvanitakis M, Dumonceau JM, Barthet M, Saunders B, Turino SY, Dhillon A, Fragaki M, Gonzalez JM, Repici A, van Wanrooij RLJ, van Hooft JE. Diagnosis and management of iatrogenic endoscopic perforations: European Society of Gastrointestinal Endoscopy (ESGE) Position Statement - Update 2020. Endoscopy. 2020 Sep;52(9):792-810.

[27] Le Greves SS, Bremseth PL, Biagini M, Holst R, Qvist N. Effect of postoperative diclofenac on anastomotic strength and histologic healing in rabbit small intestine. Int Surg. 2015;100(11):1435-42.

[28] Mayhew D, Mendonca V, Murthy BVS. A review of ASA physical status – historical perspectives and modern developments. Anaesthesia. 2019;74(3):373-9.

[29] O'Donnell M, Weitz JI. Thromboprophylaxis in surgical patients. Can J Surg. 2003;46(2):129-35.

[30] Mandalà V, editor. The Role of Laparoscopy in Emergency Abdominal Surgery. Milano: Springer Milan; 2012. (Updates in Surgery).

[31] Agresta F, Ansaloni L, Baiocchi GL, Bergamini C, Campanile FC, Carlucci M, et al. Laparoscopic approach to acute abdomen from the consensus development conference of the Società Italiana di Chirurgia Endoscopica e nuove tecnologie (SICE), Associazione Chirurghi Ospedalieri Italiani (ACOI), Società Italiana di Chirurgia (SIC), Società Italiana di Chirurgia d'Urgenza e del Trauma (SICUT), Società Italiana di Chirurgia nell'Ospedalità. Surg Endosc. 2012;26(8):2134-64.

[32] Afaque, M.Y., Alam, J., Riyaz, M. et al. Small Bowel Anastomosis Single-Layer Close Suturing—Open-Label Case Series. Indian J Surg 2020. https://doi.org/10.1007/s12262-020-02479-2